Ambulance Aid

Ambulance Aid

Nich Woolf AASI
Station Manager, Somerset Ambulance Service

Glynn Laverack RGN, NDN Cert
Clinical Nurse Manager, Frenchay Hospital, Bristol

with a foreword by
R. Snook MD FETC

Baillière Tindall
London Philadelphia
Toronto Sydney Tokyo

Baillière Tindall   24–28 Oval Road
    WB Saunders   London NW1 7DX, England

West Washington Square
Philadelphia, PA 19105, USA

1 Goldthorne Avenue
Toronto, Ontario M8Z 5T9, Canada

ABP Australia Ltd, 44–50 Waterloo Road
North Ryde, NSW 2113, Australia

Harcourt Brace Jovanovich Japan Inc.
Ichibancho Central Building, 22–1 Ichibancho
Chiyoda-ku, Tokyo 102, Japan

First published 1987

Typeset by Photo-graphics, Honiton, Devon
Printed and bound in Great Britain by
Biddles Ltd, Guildford and King's Lynn

British Library Cataloguing in Publication Data

Woolf, Nich
    Ambulance aid.
    1. First aid in illness and injury
    2. Ambulance service
    I. Title II. Laverack, Glynn
    616.02'52   RC86.7

    ISBN 0–7020–1246–7

Contents

Foreword

A period of rapid technological growth such as we are currently experiencing leads to an increase in the standards of practice at work. This in turn creates a corresponding increase in the need for information and continuing education.

Developments are taking place at such a rapid pace that all professionals have to continue the assimilation of knowledge in their field to the point of retirement. This building of knowledge is all the more secure if based on an understanding of the key factors in the subject. There is therefore a place for the soundly based standard work on a subject, and the value of such a publication is greatly enhanced if it includes the experience of application.

The authors of this book have joined to form a complementary partnership, the one actively involved in the practical implementation of the subject and the other offering the experience of a career extending from ambulance aid to hospital nursing. The result of this collaboration has been to create a blend of theory and practice. Nowhere is this more important than in the field of ambulance aid, a branch of health-care that has seen tremendous changes in the last two decades—from simple first aid to sophisticated resuscitation. All of these advances need an in-depth understanding of patient care. Emergencies are in essence a destabilization of life's systems. Instability needs careful handling to preserve and restore the balance; therefore the necessary restorative skills must be based on a confidence in the subject that will allow rapid decisions to be made in response to the situation.

Once the emergency has been stabilized the patient has to be delivered to the hospital for further care. This demands an understanding of the procedures for communicating in a common language with the other health-care professionals—a language that encompasses such common terms as patterns of injury, procedures performed, drugs given, responses seen and observations recorded. When ambulance staff converse with the receiving nurse or doctor in the same terms the transfer of vital information is ensured and the patient's care continues without interruption. This is the true measure of integration and understanding.

The aim of this book is to offer ambulance staff the resource with which to build that secure understanding of the subject for the patient's sake.

DR R. SNOOK MD FETC
Consultant in Accident
and Emergency Medicine

Preface

Since the 1960s the training of ambulance personnel has progressed slowly on a path that has led on from basic first aid towards today's extended training. To those involved ambulance aid has been, without doubt, a real subject in its own right. Others, even those in the health services, have not always considered ambulance aid to be anything but a branch of their own fields.

When we started to write this book we were each at the business end of handling casualties, one engaged in front-line ambulance work, the other in an intensive care unit. This book is intended to be for ambulance personnel and is written by people who have got their hands dirty in practical situations.

There are many worthy books on immediate care. However, few are intended specifically for ambulance personnel. Even fewer are written exclusively by people who have experience of the working environment.

Research in medicine is often hospital-based. Thus, ambulance aid has developed without the benefit of a large body of research. Much research work awaits anyone with the ability and opportunity to carry it out. There is the exciting prospect, therefore, of radical developments in the subject.

Putting our heads above the parapet we fully expect to get shot at. Hopefully some of the bullets will be constructive and thereby will make a real contribution to the subject of ambulance aid.

NICH WOOLF
GLYNN LAVERACK

For all the happiness mankind can gain
Is not in pleasure, but in rest from pain.

The Hind and the Panther — Dryden

Acknowledgements

As this title progressed from an idea to its present form, a huge number of people played a part in providing encouragement and comment.

Without David Dickens, pen would never have reached paper. Doctors Roger Snook and Peter Baskett ensured that we kept on the straight and narrow whilst still permitting originality. We are extremely grateful to Dr Snook for writing the foreword.

Jill Weymont, Bill Gardner, Len Lord and Brian Finnagan put up with being pestered about dates and wrote the chapters where we lacked expertise. They all doubted their ability to do the business but came up trumps.

Baillière Tindall, first in the form of Graham Smith and later Jeannie Labno, have given us the back-up that only a professional medical publisher can.

Thanks are due to the many friends who have read the manuscript, corrected spelling and helped with research.

Rachel, Ann, Ben and Emma, in stoic family tradition, endured the long hours of loneliness that go with shift-work and writing.

1

The Patient

AMBULANCE AID

Ambulance aid is the role of ambulance personnel. It includes the skills of getting to the patient, diagnosing his or her ailments, immediate treatment, transport to the most appropriate place for further treatment and an accurate and full handover of information to medical staff.

THE PATIENT AS A WHOLE

In addition to the abilities of diagnosis and treatment ambulance personnel must be able to obtain information and pass it on accurately when the patient is handed over. To do this requires a good knowledge of anatomy and physiology and the ability to gain the confidence of the patient. Descriptions of signs and symptoms must be:

- Concise—time may be precious
- Clear—misunderstanding could prove fatal
- Comprehensive—everything has a meaning

Written information may be superior to spoken communication. It can be checked over and received accurately long after it is written (for use of charts see chapter 4).

Terms used in anatomy

To standardize description a number of terms are used to describe the human body (Fig. 1.1).

Anatomical position. The patient standing erect facing the observer, arms beside the body, palms turned forward.

Right and left.   Refer to the patient's right and left sides opposite to those of the observer.

Median line.   An imaginary line that divides the left and right side of the patient's body.

1

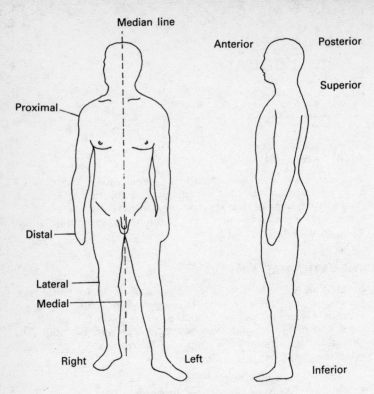

Fig. 1.1 Terms used in anatomy.

Medial. Towards the median line.

Lateral. Towards the side, away from the mid-line.

Anterior and posterior. Front and back of the patient respectively.

Superior and inferior. Towards the head or above — superior; towards the feet or below — inferior.

Proximal and distal. Closer to and further from a specified point.

Structure of the body

The basic unit of organization of the human body is the cell. There are many different types of cells, each type having specialist functions within the body.

Groups of cells form tissues, of which there are five basic types:

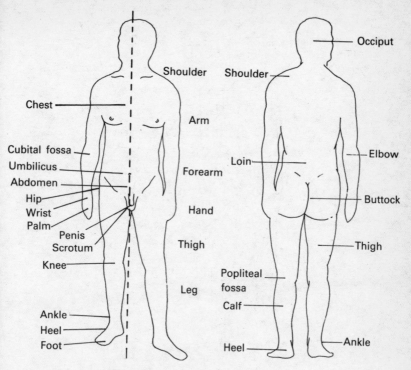

Fig. 1.2 External features of the body.

- Epithelial
- Connective
- Nervous
- Muscular
- Blood

A collection of tissues carrying out a specialist function is known as an organ.

A group of organs carrying out a specific function is a system. The main systems of the body are:

- Respiratory—exchange of gases for cell function
- Circulatory—transport of gases, foodstuff and waste products
- Skeletal—support and protection
- Muscular—movement
- Digestive—breakdown and absorption
- Urinary—excretion and metabolic balance

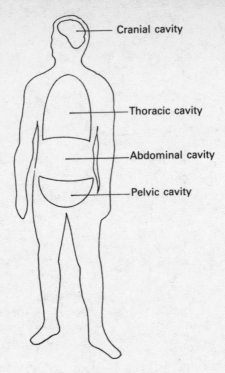

Fig. 1.3 The major body cavities.

- Nervous—control and awareness
- Endocrine—production of hormones
- Reproductive—survival of the species
- Integumentary—containment of the body

COMMUNICATION

Communication is a two-way process. It involves talking, listening and non-verbal means. In addition it involves a continuous process of feedback to check that information has been correctly passed.

Without communication ambulance aid does not take place. In the course of an emergency call, communication takes place at a number of levels:

- Patient or those around him call for an ambulance.
- Appropriate vehicle is sent to the incident.
- Crew gather information and history.
- Reassurance is provided to the patient and others.
- Information is relayed to hospital.
- Patient is informed of the treatment to be given.
- Further information is gathered during the journey.
- Information is handed over at hospital.

Since communication forms such a central part of ambulance aid it should be considered an essential skill. Some people appear to be better at communicating than others but this does not mean that these skills cannot be learnt.

In an emergency almost all patients will be under stress. In addition ambulance personnel, as strangers, may meet resistance to communication, especially of private details. It is not possible to give exact guidance on how to overcome these problems. However the following points will help:

- The use of jargon confuses both patients and medical staff.
- Some words have no precise meaning. If used they must be qualified. For example the word 'normal' means little to a stranger until it is backed up with details.
- Obtain confirmation that you have been understood.
- Use non-verbal means to assist communication. Steady eye contact and being at the same level as the patient will reassure the patient.
- Be positive and encouraging but do not dismiss the patient's problems.
- Remember that patients have the right to run their own lives. Do not judge them.

Reassurance

Of all forms of communication reassurance is the most difficult to carry out successfully. In most cases the patient is going through an experience that ambulance personnel have not had. Reassurance is an essential part of treatment, not only of the patient but also of friends and relatives.

Reassurance must be positive, showing:

- That everything possible is being done.
- What will happen next, dispelling fear of the unknown.

Remember that false reassurance will always be found out.

2

Skeleton, Muscles and Joints

ANATOMY

There are more than 200 bones in the body. To effectively treat
injury to the skeletal system it is necessary to understand the
anatomy, likely injury sites and the surrounding structures that
may be damaged.

Periosteum

The periosteum covers all but the bearing surfaces of bones. Its
function is to provide blood vessels and nerves to the bone. In
addition it provides attachment for tendons. If the periosteum is
damaged the bone may die.

Development of bones

Bones develop from centres of ossification. Figure 2.1 shows a
typical long bone. Increase in length occurs by growth of the
diaphysis from the epiphyseal cartilages until the ages of between
18 and 25 years. A fracture close to the epiphysis of a growing
bone may stop further growth.

Head and face

Any injury to the head or face may cause damage to the nervous
system and the neck (see chapter 4). There are a large number of
openings in the skull for the passage of blood vessels and nerves.
Fractures running across these openings may cause blood and/or
cerebrospinal fluid to issue from the ears, nose or mouth. Figure
2.2 shows the bones of the orbit. A blow to the cheek may fracture
some of these bones, causing an alteration of the position of the
eyes. In rare cases the contents of the orbit become trapped in the
fracture. This is termed a blow-out fracture. The only movable
joint of the head — the temporomandibular joint — is often
dislocated.

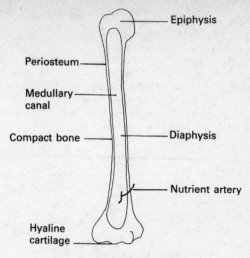

Fig. 2.1 A typical long bone.

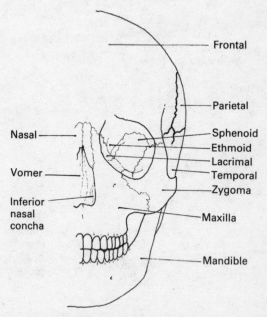

Fig. 2.2 The bones of the orbit.

Spine

The spinal column is composed of 33 bones held together as a semi-rigid structure by a large number of ligaments, tendons and muscles. Fractures may be of any of the processes or of the body (Fig. 2.3). The spinal cord fills the neural canal down to the first lumbar vertebra. The nerves of the cauda equina are closely associated with the spine for the remainder of its length. The structures affected by damage to the cord at any particular level are dealt with in chapter 4.

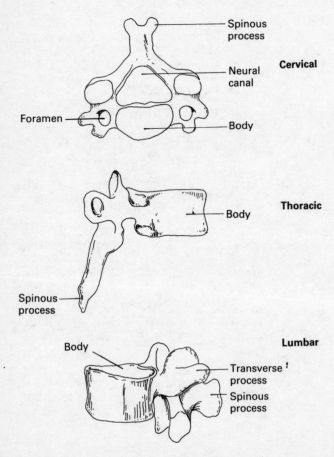

Fig. 2.3 Typical vertebrae.

Trunk

The bones of the trunk include the shoulder girdle, the ribs, the sternum, the costal cartilages and the pelvis. Figure 2.4 shows the common injury sites. Bones of the trunk surround vital organs, so complications are always a possibility in the event of a fracture.

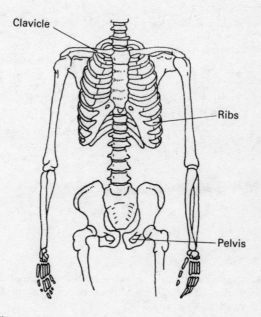

Fig. 2.4 Common injury sites—bones of the trunk.

Limbs

The close association of blood vessels and nerves with limb bones, and the shortening caused by muscle action, cause a risk of complications. Figure 2.5 shows the major blood vessels and nerves in relation to the bones of the limbs. Figure 2.6 shows the common sites of fracture and dislocation. The close association of nerves and blood vessels in the joints means that dislocation frequently causes damage to structures. The labrum may also be damaged, predisposing to a repeat dislocation.

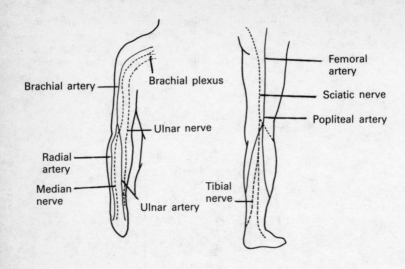

Fig. 2.5   Major blood vessels and nerves of the limbs.

DIAGNOSIS

A working diagnosis must be made before treatment. If in doubt the more serious condition must be assumed. Among the injuries that can be diagnosed are:

- Fracture—discontinuity of the bone surface
- Dislocation—displacement of bones in a joint
- Sprain—injury of joint ligaments
- Strain—muscle injury by stretching

Signs and symptoms of fractures

- **History** of direct or indirect force sufficient to fracture bone.
- **Pain** in the region of the injury, made worse by any attempt at movement.
- **Tenderness** when pressure is applied to the injury site.
- **Swelling**, immediate or delayed.
- **Deformity** may be seen as angulation at the fracture site, rotation of a limb or shortening.

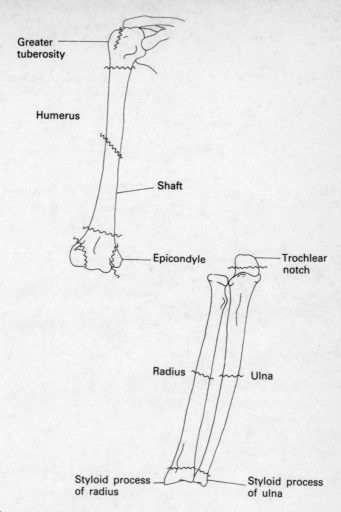

Fig. 2.6a Common sites of fracture and dislocation of the upper limb.

- **Loss of function,** i.e. inability to move the affected part or to bear weight.
- **Unnatural movement** where attempts at movement produce result other than at the joints.
- **Crepitus,** the sound or feeling of grating bone.
- **Lack of feeling,** loss of sensation distal to the injury site.

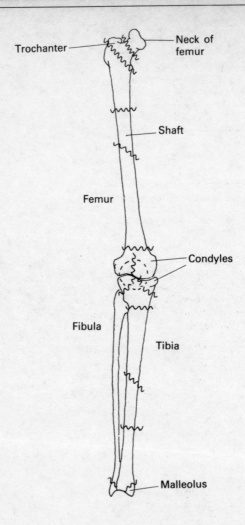

Fig. 2.6b Common sites of fracture and dislocation of the lower limb.

Most fractures will display only some of the signs and symptoms. Without the benefit of radiography any two of the signs and symptoms occurring together should indicate a possible fracture.

Signs and symptoms of joint injuries

- Dislocation—signs and symptoms as fractures but with pain and tenderness centred on a joint. The joint is often fixed. A dislocated joint has a different overall shape; bone ends may be prominent under the skin.
- Sprains—pain, tenderness, loss of power and swelling of the joint. The history will show a movement that stretched the ligaments of the affected joint.
- Contusions—swelling and inability to move the joint. History will show a direct blow to a joint followed by swelling after several hours.
- Internal disruption—signs and symptoms similar to a dislocation but without the displacement of bones.

Testing the skeleton

In an unconscious patient active movements can only be checked if the patient happens to make them. With a conscious patient some of these steps will be superfluous where injury is obvious. The examination proceeds in a set order so as to find the most important injuries first. Many elderly patients will not have the full range of movements. For examination of the unconscious patient, see chapter 4.

Movement of the joints. Joints can move in six possible ways:

- Flexion—bending
- Extension—straightening
- Abduction—moving away from the median line
- Adduction—moving towards the median line
- Rotation (internal and external)—turning in or out
- Circumduction—combining all movements in a circular motion

In addition there are non-movable joints such as the facial and cranial bones, and slightly movable joints such as the symphysis pubis.

Testing the neck and head. On approaching the patient look for a history that could suggest a neck injury. If the patient has no pain in the neck, press firmly on each cervical vertebra, feeling for displacement and asking if there is tenderness.

If nothing is found or felt the patient should be asked to extend and rotate the neck. This should be followed by left and right lateral flexion.

The head should be felt all over, gently checking especially the nasal bones and zygomatic arches. Open the mouth and look inside, close the jaw and check movement from side to side.

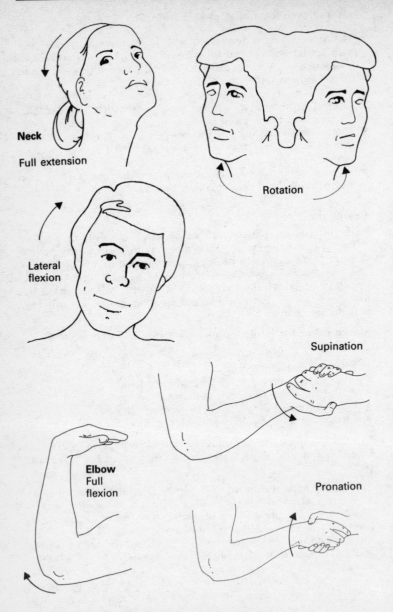

Neck

Full extension

Rotation

Lateral
flexion

Supination

Elbow
Full
flexion

Pronation

Fig. 2.7 Movement of the joints.

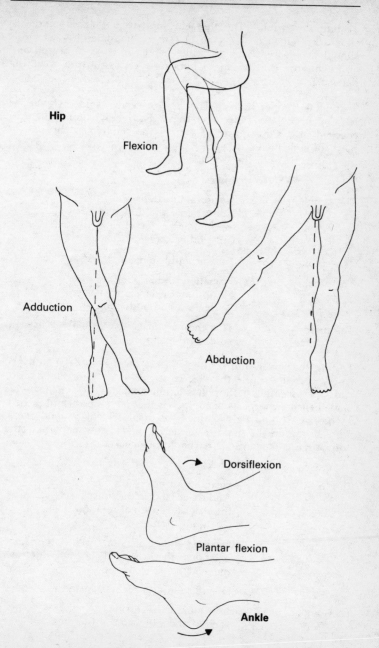

Hip

Flexion

Adduction

Abduction

Dorsiflexion

Plantar flexion

Ankle

Testing the trunk. The thoracic, lumbar and sacral vertebrae should be felt to find any displacement or tenderness. The ribs should be pressed by placing the hands under each armpit and also gently on the sternum. Check for a change in the breathing pattern.

Testing the upper limbs. The clavicles and scapulae should be felt for irregularity and tenderness. Each arm should then be checked in a similar way. If there is no tenderness the normal range of movements for each joint should be checked, comparing the right side with the left side.

Check:

The shoulder	Flexion and extension
	Abduction and adduction
	Internal and external rotation
	Circumduction
The elbow	Flexion and extension
The wrist	Pronation and supination
	Flexion and extension
	Abduction and adduction
The hand	That the patient is able to make a fist and spread his palm

Testing the lower limbs. Press firmly on the pubic symphysis. Apply pressure across the iliac crests. Press on both the anterior and superior spines of the pelvis simultaneously. These manoeuvres may elicit pain in parts of the pelvis that have not been touched.

The legs should be examined for displacement or tenderness. Press firmly on the great trocanter. If there is no tenderness the normal range of movements should be checked.

Check:

The hip	Flexion and extension
	Abduction and adduction
	Internal and external rotation
	Circumduction
The knee	Flexion and extension. With the knee extended there should be no sideways movement.
The ankle	Dorsiflexion and plantar flexion
The foot	Inversion and eversion
	Flexion and extension of the toes

Mechanism of injury

Fractures are caused:

- By direct force—a sharp blow or heavy weight. Some bones such as the skull are normally broken only by direct force.
- By indirect force—the force is transmitted along bones to fracture at a distant site. The clavicle is commonly fractured by a fall on the outstretched arm. The base of the skull may be fractured by a heavy landing on the heels.
- By muscle action—a sudden jerk may cause fractures. This is commonly seen with a kick that misses the ball.
- For pathological reasons—the bone is so weakened by disease, especially secondary carcinoma, that any movement may give rise to a fracture.

Joint injuries are caused by:

- Dislocation—a pull or levering action working out from the joint.
- Sprains—stretching or rupturing the ligaments that hold a joint together.
- Contusions—a blow causing an effusion into a joint.
- Internal disruption—twisting a joint in a way in which it is not designed to move. This is most commonly seen in twisting of the knee, displacing the menisci.

Classification of fractures

- Closed—the skin is intact.
- Open—the skin is damaged, allowing communication with the fracture. This may lead to the entrance of infection. Foreign matter trapped in the lumen of a long bone is a common cause of malunion. Severe angulation may lead to the bone end becoming contaminated outside the limb. The bone end may or may not have re-entered the limb before examination.
- Complicated—the broken bone has damaged other structures. Common complications are damaged blood vessels and nerves. Other complications are punctured lung or liver and laceration of the brain by skull fragments.
- Impacted—one fractured end becomes lodged inside the other. The limb may appear stable but will be shortened.
- Pathological—the bone fractures at a line of weakness. This is usually due to disease or old age.
- Greenstick—although the overall shape of the bone has been altered it has not broken into pieces. The periosteum is usually intact. This is usually found in children.

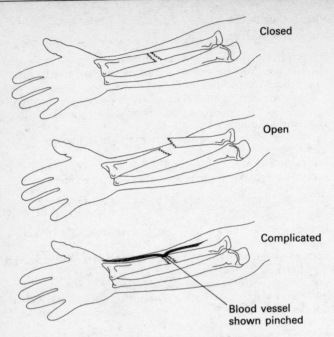

Fig. 2.8   The classification of fractures.

Diagnosis of complications

For any fracture three types of complication must be looked for: complications of blood vessels, nerves and other organs. In this context the skin is an important organ of the body.

Where limbs have been fractured, sensation and pulse must be checked distal to the fracture. If a pulse cannot be found the perfusion of the nail beds gives some indication of the quality of circulation. In addition a limb lacking circulation will be cold.

Even if a pulse is present in a limb the skin may be deprived of circulation. This may be because of pressure by a displaced bone end or necrosis caused by tagging of the skin (Fig. 2.11).

Where organs may have been damaged as a result of fractures the appropriate tests should be made. Examples of organ damage signs and symptoms are: the desire to micturate following a pelvic fracture, deep shock following puncture of the spleen by a fractured rib, and blood in the urine caused by a fractured rib damaging a kidney.

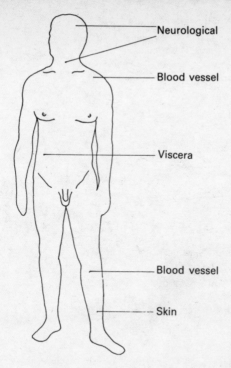

Fig. 2.9 Complications of fractures.

Diagnosis of specific injuries

Certain fractures, because of their special nature or common occurrence, have characteristic signs and symptoms. Some need special safeguards to be taken as soon as they have been diagnosed.

Skull fractures.   A force large enough to fracture bones in the head is sufficient to damage the cervical vertebrae. Thus if a skull fracture is suspected the neck should be assessed and safeguarded as appropriate. Some skull fractures are depressed. When feeling the surface of the cranium the touch must be gentle to avoid pressing bone fragments into the brain. Especially in children, skull fracture may be like broken eggshell; small fragments of bone are held in place by skin but in reality this is a depressed fracture.

Fracture of the base of skull may allow blood and/or cerebrospinal fluid to issue from the nose, mouth and ears. (See also chapter 4 for examination of the unconscious patient.)

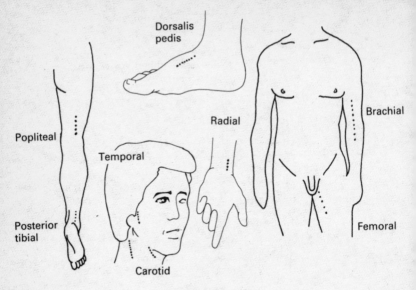

Fig. 2.10 Pulse sites.

Spinal fractures. There may be displacement of vertebrae, in which case the cord is at risk of damage. A vertebra may have collapsed or there may be an unstable fracture (Fig. 2.12).

Diagnosis is made from history, pain at injury site, loss of feeling and/or power in the limbs and the patient saying that he feels 'cut in half'. A persistent erection—priapism—is a sign of cord damage. (See also examination of the unconscious patient, chapter 4.)

Fractures of the wrist. The distal end of the radius is commonly fractured by a fall on the outstretched hand. A Colles' fracture is an extension fracture of the wrist showing the so-called dinner fork deformity. The similar fracture with the wrist flexed showing flexion deformity is called a Smith's fracture (Fig. 2.13).

Fractures of the ankle. The talus sits between the malleoli, and a twisting force will lever the mortice joint open, fracturing one, two or even three of the medial, lateral or posterior malleoli. This is commonly referred to as a Pott's fracture (Fig. 2.14).

Injury to the neck of the femur. This is common in the elderly. The leg is shortened and the foot is turned outward. Pain may be

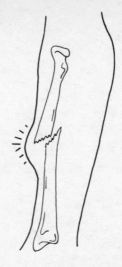

Fig. 2.11   Necrosis caused by tagging of the skin.

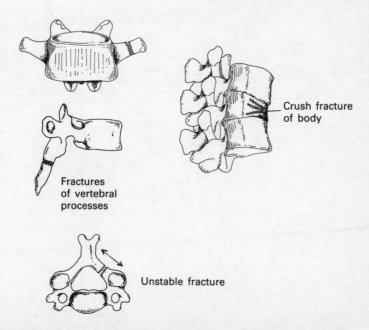

Crush fracture
of body

Fractures
of vertebral
processes

Unstable fracture

Fig. 2.12   The displacement, collapse and unstable fracture of vertebrae.

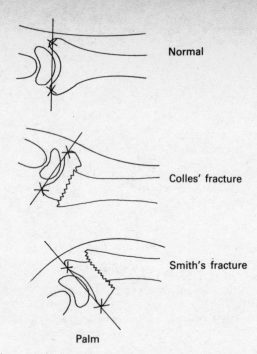

Normal

Colles' fracture

Smith's fracture

Palm

Fig. 2.13 Colles' and Smith's fractures of the wrist.

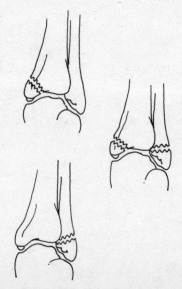

Fig. 2.14 Fractures of the ankle.

minimal. In the elderly the history may be of only a very slight force causing the fracture.

Dislocation of the humerus. This may be caused by a fall or pull. The head of the humerus may be anterior or posterior to the socket. In anterior dislocation comparison with the good shoulder will show a difference and the head of the humerus can be seen.

Dislocation of the hip. This is often associated with other injuries due to the great force necessary to dislocate such a large joint. Dislocation may be posterior or anterior. Posterior dislocation may be accompanied by a fracture of the margin of the acetabulum. Signs are shortening, internal rotation and slight flexion of the knee.

TREATMENT

Principles of treatment

- A clear airway and good circulation must be assured before the treatment of fractures (see chapter 3).
- Reassurance must be given and, in the conscious patient, confidence must be gained.
- Multiple fractures and complications must be sought.
- The entry of dirt or contamination into open fractures must be prevented or limited.
- The patient should be made comfortable and measures taken to relieve pain.
- Pain and injury must be prevented by immobilization of the affected part.
- Transport should be at a speed appropriate to the patient's condition.
- Pulse and sensation should be checked and recorded at intervals after the diagnosis of fractures.
- At hand-over of the patient a full report must be given to include history, diagnosis, changes in condition and any special circumstances.

Extrication

The patient may be trapped or may have fallen into a confined space. Even a patient lying in the open may be in circumstances that do not allow full diagnosis and treatment before moving. Each situation will present its own set of problems. To minimize further damage the patient must be lifted with the maximum of support and the minimum disturbance to position of limbs. This may entail the use of a carry sheet, canvas, poles and spreaders, or an orthopaedic, Neil Robertson or Paraguard stretcher.

Where an acutely angulated limb must be straightened to remove the patient from an obstruction the bone ends must move as little as possible. Movement must be gentle, steady and planned. Gentle but strong traction will be required but must not be released until the limb is immobilized in the extended position.

Where there is a crush injury the existence of penetrating wounds must be investigated before removal. See chapter 3.

Splints and splinting

- Support must extend past the joint above and below the fracture site.
- Open wounds must be dressed before splinting.
- Skin-to-skin contact must be padded to avoid chafing or pressure damage.
- Splinting must be firm without impairing circulation.
- Whilst a splint is in place, circulation and sensation distal to the injury must be checked.
- Fastening should not be over the fracture site.
- The use of Entonox (see p. 132) will relax the patient and aid the application of a splint.

Types of splint

There are many different types of splint in use on ambulances. In addition there are many improvised splints. Each has advantages and disadvantages which are best learnt by practical experience. Guidelines only are given here since 'hands on' experience is the easiest way to learn. Several splints have alternative or trade names; these are shown in parentheses.

Self splints (body contour splinting). This is provided by strapping an injured limb to a good limb. Padding must be provided and the good limb must be moved to the injured limb. Self splints can be used for lower limbs, fingers and upper limbs, strapped to the trunk (Fig. 2.15).

Inflatable splints. These are usually supplied in a variety of sizes and provide firm support only for fractures distal to elbow and knee. The even pressure reduces bleeding and helps to straighten the limb. They permit continuous observation of the limb. Regular checks must be made on circulation, and pressure should be released for 5 minutes every 60 minutes (Fig. 2.16).

Box splint (Hayes splint, Frac immobilizer). Some versions of the box splint have an additional piece to keep the foot at right angles. If traction splints are not available, by fitting a wooden

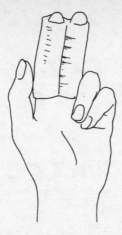

Fig. 2.15   Self-splinting one finger to another.

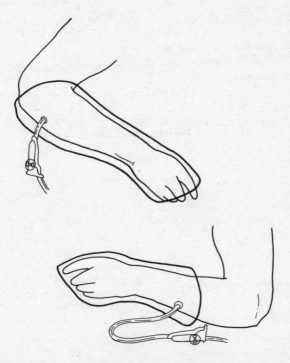

Fig. 2.16   Inflatable splints.

splint in the pocket together with a pad under the arm this splint can be used for fractures of the femur as well as of the lower leg (Fig. 2.17).

Kramer wire splint.   This is for use when limbs cannot be straightened. The wire is bent to suit the limb (Fig. 2.18).

Wooden splints.   These are fastened with triangular bandages or Frac straps to form an effective splint, but must be well padded to protect the skin (Fig. 2.19).

Short spinal board.   This is fitted to the patient in situ before removal. It is mainly used for cervical fractures. There are now a variety of alternatives serving the same purpose. Careful practice is essential before use. As with all spinal injuries there is no replacement for slow, careful and preplanned handling (Fig. 2.20).

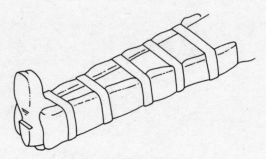

Fig. 2.17   Box splint.

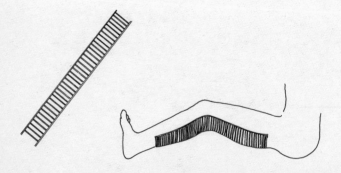

Fig. 2.18   Kramer wire splint.

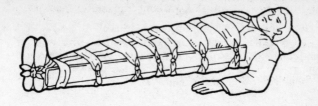

Fig. 2.19 Wooden splints for a fractured femur.

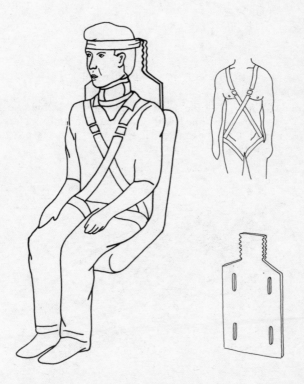

Fig. 2.20 Short spinal board.

Cervical collar. A range of sizes is required. It may be used with or without a short spinal board, but it must not constrict the neck.

Traction splints. Several different kinds are in use, each of which needs special practical training before use. The principle is to counteract the muscular action, relieve pain and prevent further damage. Padding presses on the ischial tuberosity whilst tension is applied to the malleoli (Fig. 2.21).

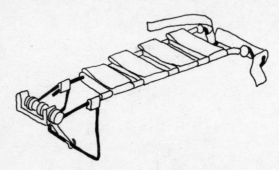

Fig. 2.21 A Hare traction splint.

Vacuum splints. Ranging from whole body to individual limb splints, these are bags filled with granules. The limb is placed on the splint and the air is extracted. The granules are packed together and the splint becomes rigid (Fig. 2.22).

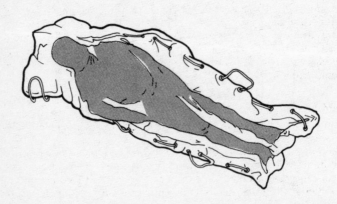

Fig. 2.22 A vacuum splint.

Blanket splints.   The various blanket folds taught in basic training can provide excellent splints, especially for limbs outside the normal size range (Fig. 2.23).

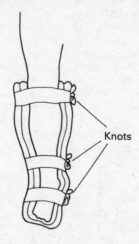

Knots

Fig. 2.23   A blanket splint.

Transport

Ambulance transport must suit the condition of the patient. Fractures will impose a slow speed and smooth ride on the driver. In the case of uncomplicated spinal injuries a smooth ride is required above all other considerations. Acute blood loss would appear to call for a faster journey to hospital. However, if the immobilization is not sufficient, blood loss will be aggravated by a rough ride.

Blood loss

Blood loss may be from the bone and periosteum, damaged muscles or damaged blood vessels.

Blood loss may cause swelling of a limb in a closed fracture or may be lost from an open fracture. Fractures of bones such as the pelvis can cause blood loss into body cavities with little external sign. Blood loss from open fractures must be controlled by pressure around the wound, which must be padded so as not to press on bone ends (see chapter 3).

Fractures of the head and face

The airway is at risk not only from neurological complications but also from blood, cerebrospinal fluid, vomit and the displacement of false teeth or the tongue. The mandible is the only bone that may need immobilization, but because of the risk of airway obstruction this is only possible in the fully conscious patient capable of maintaining his own airway.

With maxillofacial injuries the swelling of soft tissues is considerable. This makes accurate reporting important since fracture sites may be masked by swelling within a few minutes. The patient may be unable to speak due to the injuries. This will create anxiety as well as hindering diagnosis.

Reassurance will be needed for both conscious and unconscious patients. False teeth, even if broken, can form a valuable record of the shape of a patient's face in fractures of the maxilla. Real or false teeth may come loose following injury and lodge in the respiratory tract.

Fractures close to the orbit of the eye may interfere with vision by displacing one eye relative to the other.

If conscious and able to maintain a good airway, the patient may be transported in a semi-recumbent position. More normally a patient with an impaired level of consciousness must be either intubated or conveyed in the recovery position with suction used to clear the airway. Alternatively, Figure 2.24 shows blanket pads used to provide a drainage position. Special care must be taken of the neck in fractures of the head and face since the forces involved may be sufficient to also cause cervical damage. Patients

Blanket with two folded portions — one at forehead level and one at chest level

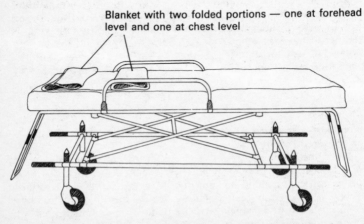

Fig. 2.24 A stretcher with blanket pads for maxillofacial injuries.

reporting pain or tenderness in the cervical region and all unconscious patients should have a cervical collar applied.

Limb injuries

Treatment must be of the whole limb. The injury may be a fracture of the bone but the other structures of the limb are also important. Movement of the bone ends may damage muscle or blood vessels. Pressure by bone ends or external sources may damage the skin, causing treatment in hospital to be prolonged and infection to enter the limb.

The muscle of the limb often causes shortening. This is especially common in fractures of the femur. It should be managed by splinting with gentle countertraction.

No attempt should be made to manipulate a dislocation. Instead the limb should be immobilized in a position comfortable to the patient.

Sprains are often difficult to distinguish from fractures, so they should be treated in the same way as a fracture if there is any doubt.

Pelvic injuries

Because the pelvis is full of important organs there is a high risk of complications. Immobilization is carried out in two phases (Fig. 2.25). First, the pelvis is bound around so that any fractures are held closed. Second, the legs are held together, slightly flexed for comfort, to prevent leverage on the sides of the pelvis. The patient may have the urge to micturate but should be told to resist since the integrity of the bladder and urethra is in doubt. This will cause considerable anxiety which must be counteracted by reassurance. If the patient has passed urine the presence or absence of blood should be checked.

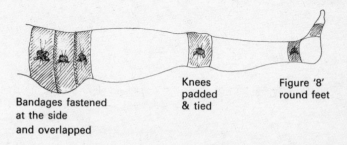

Bandages fastened
at the side
and overlapped

Knees
padded
& tied

Figure '8'
round feet

Fig. 2.25 Immobilization of the pelvis.

The pelvis is in the form of a ring. It may be fractured in one place, leaving it relatively stable. With two fractures there may be no effective connection between the hips.

Spinal injuries

Spinal injuries differ considerably in severity. The treatment, however, must be comprehensive in all suspected cases. Especially in cases of high cervical lesions signs of change should be watched for carefully. Oedema of the cord may cause gradual neurological damage (see chapter 4).

Entonox should not be given until splinting and immobilization are complete.

A methodical approach is essential. Reassurance is required at all stages and the patient must be kept informed of all the actions to be carried out.

Space must be cleared around the patient in preparation for lifting. The lift must be planned so that the patient is transferred onto a structure such as a canvas or orthopaedic stretcher in one step. Thereafter all handling is of this structure, with the patient remaining immobile.

All helpers must be briefed before lifting or carrying. There is only one opportunity to get such manoeuvres right.

Loading and transport must be smooth. This will necessitate a slow speed, the avoidance of bumps and careful cornering, and acceleration and braking must be kept to a minimum.

At hospital, nursing staff should be briefed about the patient before his transfer to hospital equipment.

Cervical injuries can be treated with a short spinal board and a cervical collar (Fig. 2.20). Injuries lower down the spine must be immobilized and lifted by orthopaedic stretcher (Fig. 2.26) or canvas and poles.

For transport, the natural curves of the spine can be supported by spinal pads (Fig. 2.27). Sandbags should be used to prevent side-to-side movement.

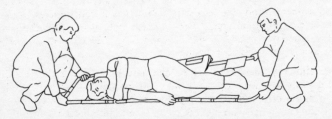

Fig. 2.26   An orthopaedic (scoop) stretcher.

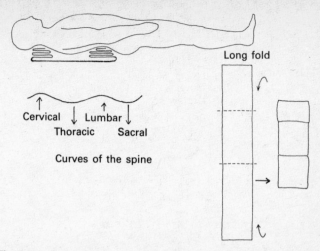

Long fold

Cervical   Lumbar
Thoracic   Sacral

Curves of the spine

Fig. 2.27 The position of blanket pads on stretcher for spinal injury.

Peripheral sensation and motor function of the fingers and toes must be tested at regular intervals and any changes reported on arrival at hospital.

Fractures of the ribs and sternum

Pain relief and good positioning is the only treatment possible. There is a considerable risk of complications (see chapter 3).

Fractures of the lower limb

Femur. In the elderly patient a fracture of the femur may be painless, caused by something as simple as a stumble or rolling over in bed. This will require strapping the good leg to the fractured leg followed by careful handling (Fig. 2.28). The patient should be placed in a position that is comfortable to him.

In other age groups a fracture of the femur is usually the result of more serious trauma and is associated with great pain. Shortening often takes place by as much as 10 centimetres. Fractures near the popliteal space carry a great risk of complications. Both hip and knee must be immobilized (Fig. 2.29). Traction splinting, if available, is advantageous.

Patella. A fracture of the patella may be caused either by direct force or by muscular action. The patient is often unable to straighten the knee. A long wooden splint is ideal since the space under the knee can be accurately padded to give support (Fig. 2.30).

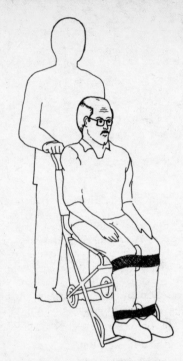

Fig. 2.28 Treatment of an elderly patient with a fractured femur.

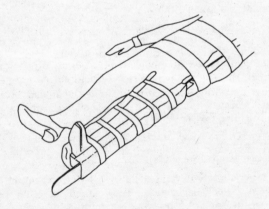

Fig. 2.29 Treatment of a fractured femur in a young adult.

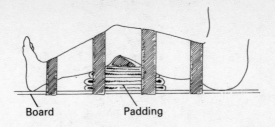

Fig. 2.30 Splinting of a fractured patella.

Lower leg. A fracture to the lower leg is usually caused by direct force. The tibia is situated close to the skin, and direct force often creates an open fracture. This may well be associated with road dirt or mud. If boots are removed, blood loss may be aggravated. Inflatable splints may be used, but for complicated or open fractures a box splint allows easier access during transport. The foot should be supported at 90° and in line with the knee (Fig. 2.17).

Ankle and foot. The distinction between a sprain and a fracture of the ankle and foot is not possible without X-rays in many cases. Splinting and support on a folded blanket will provide comfort (Fig. 2.23).

Fractures of the upper limb

Clavicle. This is most often fractured by indirect force, e.g. a fall on an outstretched arm. The shoulder drops forward. The patient will normally support his own arm in a comfortable position. Support can be assisted by a triangular sling with a pad under the arm (Fig. 2.31).

Scapula. This is almost always fractured by direct force. Ribs underneath the scapula may also be fractured. A large arm sling will take the weight of the arm and provide some comfort.

Humerus. Fractures of the proximal end of the humerus usually occur across the surgical neck or at the base of the greater tuberosity. The fracture may be impacted. Fractures of the distal half carry a greater risk of complications. If movement of the elbow is not affected a large arm sling will give support. If the elbow cannot be bent the arm can be splinted to the body and the patient transported lying flat.

Elbow. Fractures close to the elbow often result in pieces of bone being pulled out of position. There is a risk of complications and the position of the joint should not be moved.

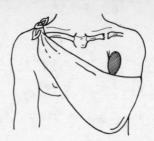

Sling & pad under arm
Ends of clavicle held apart

Fig. 2.31   A triangular sling and pad for a fractured clavicle.

Forearm.   Fractures of the forearm may be caused by direct or indirect force and involve one or both bones. Fractures of only one bone may show little deformity. Fractures near the olecranon may leave bone fragments that have been pulled up the upper arm by muscle action. Fractures distal to the elbow are adequately dealt with by a sling or inflatable splint. A close check must be kept on circulation whilst inflatable splints are in place (Fig. 2.16).

Hand.   Fractures of the hand are almost always due to direct force. A short wooden splint with padding may be used, but most often a triangular sling will give most comfort.

3

Respiration, Circulation and Blood

An adequate supply of oxygen to the tissues is the most important aim of ambulance aid. To achieve this aim not only involves the respiratory system but also the circulatory system to deliver the oxygen. To carry out effective diagnosis and treatment it is necessary to understand the anatomy, physiology and diagnostic techniques detailed in this section.

ANATOMY AND PHYSIOLOGY OF THE RESPIRATORY AND CIRCULATORY SYSTEMS

Control of respiration

Respiration is controlled by the respiratory centre in the medulla oblongata. The vagus and glossopharyngeal nerves carry impulses to the centre from special receptors in the great arteries. These detect the level of carbon dioxide in the blood. Since carbon dioxide in solution is acid there is a direct correlation of blood pH to CO_2 level.

In some respiratory conditions such as chronic bronchitis and emphysema the patient's blood is always rich in CO_2. The respiratory centre undergoes change and becomes insensitive to CO_2 and responsive to O_2 concentration. This is called hypoxic drive.

Capacity of the lungs

The total capacity of the respiratory system in an average adult is about 5100 millilitres. Of this volume, 1100 millilitres is the residual volume. This is capacity that cannot be used. During normal respiration about 500 millilitres of air is changed with each breath. This is termed the tidal volume. After a normal tidal inspiration a further 2500 millilitres of inspiratory reserve volume can be used. Similarly, after tidal exhalation 1000 millilitres of exhalation reserve remains (Fig. 3.1).

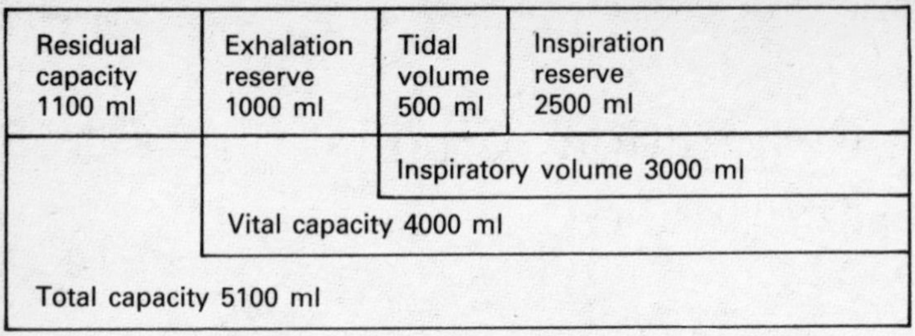

Residual capacity 1100 ml	Exhalation reserve 1000 ml	Tidal volume 500 ml	Inspiration reserve 2500 ml
		Inspiratory volume 3000 ml	
	Vital capacity 4000 ml		
Total capacity 5100 ml			

Fig. 3.1 The capacity of the lungs.

Partial pressure of gases

Air is a mixture of gases in the following proportions:

Oxygen	21%
Carbon dioxide	0.04%
Nitrogen	79%
Water vapour and rare gases	Variable

Each of these gases is responsible for a proportion of the pressure exerted by air—atmosphere pressure. This partial pressure (P) can be measured in kilopascals (kPa) or millimetres of mercury (mmHg). Gases will pass from a high to a low partial pressure if possible.

Blood volume

Total blood volume can be estimated from weight or height in adults and from age in children (Fig. 3.2a & b).

Table 1. The partial pressure exerted by various gases in different mediums.

	Alveolar air		Deoxygenated blood		Oxygenated blood	
Gas	mmHg	kPa	mmHg	kPa	mmHg	kPa
Oxygen	100	13.3	40	5.3	100	13.3
Carbon dioxide	40	5.3	44	5.8	40	5.3
Nitrogen	570	76.0	570	76.0	570	76.0
Water vapour	50	6.7				
Atmospheric pressure	760	101.3				

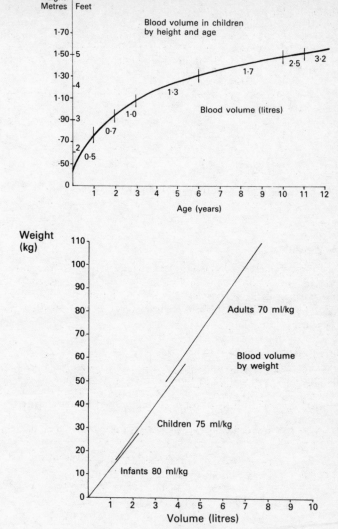

Fig. 3.2a   The estimation of blood volume.

The output of the heart is proportional to the input. A low blood volume and reduced venous return to the heart therefore reduces the output.

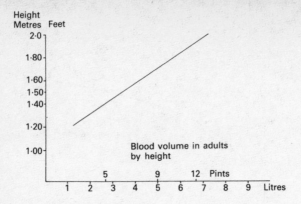

Fig. 3.2b The estimation of blood volume.

Blood pressure

Blood pressure is the force exerted on the blood vessel walls by the circulating blood. It can be altered by changes in:

- Peripheral resistance
- Elasticity of the arterial walls
- Viscosity of the blood
- Stroke volume (rate and force of the ventricles)
- Blood volume available to the heart

The pressure wave during heart contraction is called systolic pressure. Diastolic pressure is when the heart is refilling. The pressure does not drop to zero but is maintained by the elasticity of the arterial walls.

Normal blood pressure at rest is as follows:

Systolic pressure	Preschool children: 75 mmHg
	Children up to 12 years: 90 mmHg
	Teenagers: 105 mmHg
	Adult female: 90 mmHg + age
	Adult male: 100 mmHg + age
Diastolic pressure	65–90 mmHg

Composition of the blood

See Table 2.

Table 2. Composition of the blood.

Cells (comprising 45% of the blood)	Plasma (comprising 55% of the blood)
Red corpuscles (erythrocytes)	Water (90% of the blood)
Platelets (thrombocytes)	Mineral salts (0.9% of the blood)
White cells	Plasma proteins Foodstuff Gases (oxygen, carbon dioxide and nitrogen)
Granular leucocytes / Non-granular leucocytes	Waste products Antibodies Antitoxins
Baso-phil Neutro-phil Eosino-phil / Lympho-cytes Monocytes	Hormones Enzymes

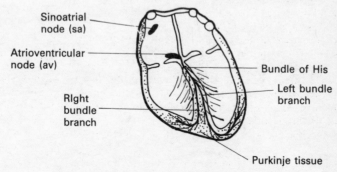

Fig. 3.3 The conducting system of the heart.

Conducting system of the heart

In health the sinoatrial node is the pacemaker of the heart under the control of the autonomic nervous system. The impulses spread across the atria, stimulating the atrioventricular node. The impulse is conducted to the ventricles by the bundle of His, the bundle branches and the Purkinje fibres (Fig. 3.3).

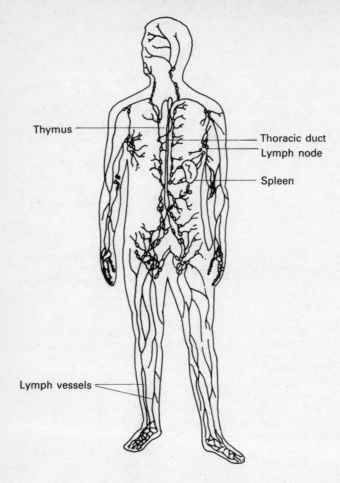

Thymus

Thoracic duct

Lymph node

Spleen

Lymph vessels

Fig. 3.4   The lymphatic system.

The lymphatic system

At the venous end of the capillaries, fluid is taken up from the interstitial space. The pressure gradient is slight and a proportion of the plasma is returned by the lymphatic system to the venous system. This consists of a series of vessels and nodes (Fig. 3.4).

DIAGNOSTIC TECHNIQUES

Pulse

Measurements can be taken at a variety of sites (Fig. 2.10). At initial examination the carotid pulse is the most reliable. In conscious patients the radial pulse is normally taken. The rate, rhythm and volume of the pulse needs to be assessed. Thus:

- What is the rate? (The rate for a newborn infant should be 140 beats/minute, whereas the rate for adults at rest should be 50–90 beats/minute.)
- Is the rhythm regular or irregular?
- Is the volume full or thready?

Measurement should be over at least 30 seconds and should be repeated. Look for evidence of drugs that may be influencing pulse rate.

Respiration

This should be assessed without the patient's knowledge. Many patients will alter their rate if they think they are being observed. Whilst taking a pulse hold the patient's wrist on their chest. The rate, rhythm, depth and nature of the respiration need to be assessed. Thus:

- What is the rate? (The rate for a child should be 25–50 respirations/minute, whereas the rate for adults should be 14–20 respirations/minute.)
- Is the rhythm regular or irregular?
- Is the depth deep or shallow?
- What is the nature?
  Normal? (quiet breathing)
  Stertorous? (snoring sounds)
  Noisy? (foreign matter or fluid in the respiratory tract)
  Cheyne–Stokes? (regular cycle of deep then shallow breathing with periods of apnoea)
  Does the chest move evenly and equally on both sides?
  Painful? (with jerky movements)

Blood pressure

Systolic pressure can be found by taking the radial pulse whilst deflating the cuff. No stethoscope is needed. This provides a good check in a noisy environment.

With an aneroid sphygmomanometer the needle can be seen to oscillate whilst between systolic and diastolic pressure. This can provide a good reading in a moving vehicle.

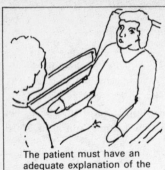

The patient must have an adequate explanation of the procedure.

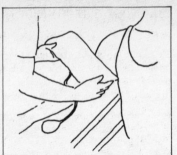

Tight clothing must be removed from the patients arm.

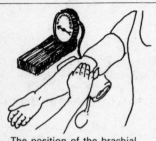

The position of the brachial artery should be established before recording commences

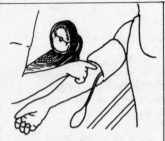

The cuff should be applied firmly. The centre of the bladder must be over the brachial artery.

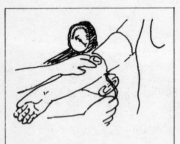

Hold the diaphragm in place with the fingers. Do not press hard.

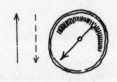

Inflation should be rapid and deflation slow (2 mm Hg/sec). After measurement break the connection for patient comfort. If pressure is missed start from the beginning.

Fig. 3.5 Taking blood pressure.

Blood pressure readings will vary for people of different sizes unless the correct size cuff is used. If the correct cuff is not available then at least a series of readings with the same cuff will give an indication of change. All blood pressure readings should be taken on the same limb (Fig. 3.5).

Use of the electrocardiogram

Specific arrhythmias are dealt with under diagnosis. Monitoring equipment varies from model to model. The electrocardiogram apparatus is activated by electrical current. The size of the wave does not indicate the strength of the heart-beat. Setting-up procedures and recognition of traces must be learnt in a practical environment (Fig. 3.6).

DIAGNOSIS

Asphyxia

Asphyxia is an insufficient supply of oxygen to the vital organs. It is caused by:

- Problems of the respiratory tract—obstruction of the airway, smothering.
- Inhibition of the respiratory centre—head injury, cerebrovascular accident, drugs, electric shock.
- Disruption of the respiratory mechanism—spinal injury, chest injuries.
- Lack of blood circulation—shock, heart disease.
- Problems of gas exchange—poisonous gases, lung disease, blast injury.
- Lack of oxygen—drowning, asphyxiant gases.

Signs of asphyxia.   These are as follows:

- History of injury or disease likely to cause asphyxia
- Dilated pupils
- Noisy breathing (if the airway is obstructed)
- Cyanosis (bluish appearance of skin and mucous membranes)
- Patient holds hand to neck

Traumatic asphyxia—compression of the chest or abdomen preventing respiration—produces:

- Petechial haemorrhages on the face
- Subconjunctival haemorrhages
- Rising blood pressure
- Falling pulse

The normal electrocardiogram

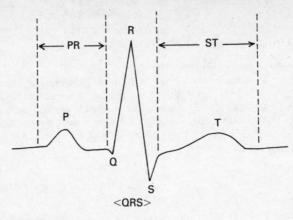

Standard times

PR	0·17–0·20 sec
ST	0·27–0·33 sec
QRS	0·08–0·10 sec

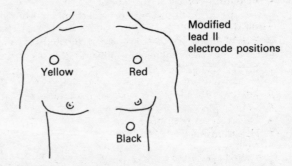

Modified lead II electrode positions

Fig. 3.6 The electrocardiogram.

Acute respiratory conditions

Obstruction. The signs and categories of obstruction are as follows:

- Obvious effort of respiration
- Noisy breathing (stertorous, stridor)
- Cyanosis

- Use of the accessory muscles of respiration
- Inadequate chest movement to inflate the lungs
- Engorged neck veins

Obstruction may be categorized into obstruction by objects, substances or swelling.

Objects

- Tongue
- Inhaled foreign body
- Teeth, broken/false/crowns

Substances

- Water
- Blood
- Vomit
- Mucus

Swelling

- Burns and scalds
- Allergic reaction
- Trauma to the throat or face
- Infectious conditions, e.g. croup

Trauma.   Trauma to the chest causes great pain. This pain, coupled with damage to the respiratory system, rapidly causes respiratory distress. All these conditions cause hypoxia.

Signs and symptoms

- History of a blow, pressure or penetration of the chest
- Pain
- Difficulty in breathing
- Haemoptysis
- Cyanosis
- Discoloration of the skin of the chest, shoulders and face, accompanied by surgical emphysema
- Distended veins in the neck
- Asymmetrical shape or movement of the chest wall
- Shock

Pneumothorax.   Air in the pleural space prevents the expansion of a lung. The air may have entered the pleural space either from damaged alveoli or from a puncture wound. The lung will collapse due to the elastic nature of its tissues.

Pneumothorax may be spontaneous, due to injury, congenital defect or disease. Wounds that penetrate the pleura may suck air in with each expansion of the chest. This is called an open pneumothorax. A tension pneumothorax is where air entering the pleural space is held in and the pressure increases due to a 'one-way valve' effect. Collapse of the lung can allow the mediastinum and the unaffected lung to be displaced.

Haemothorax.   Blood in the pleural space interferes with the normal function of the lungs. Haemothorax will cause signs of shock. Several litres of blood can potentially be lost into the pleural space.

Flail segment injuries.   Especially following crush injuries, a whole segment of the rib cage is fractured. This allows the loose part to be moved by the internal pressure differences. Paradoxical breathing, as this is known, can be seen by comparing the two sides of the chest. It is confirmed by gentle palpation, detecting bony crepitus coinciding with respiratory movement. Respiration will be inadequate and bruising of the lung will cause increasing shock.

Drowning.   Diagnosis is made from the history or circumstances. Drowning may be classified as wet, with water in the lungs, or dry. In some cases asphyxia is believed to be due to hypothermia.

Smoke inhalation.   Asphyxia may be due to poisoning, lack of oxygen or heat damage. There may be soot deposits in and around the nose and mouth. Heat may cause swelling of the tissue of the respiratory tract.

Chemical pneumonitis.   Ingestion of chemicals, especially volatile hydrocarbons such as turpentine or white spirit can cause inflammation of the lungs by inhalation or aspiration (see chapter 2).

Hyperventilation.   An agitated patient often breathes in a fast, shallow pattern. Soon, their carbon dioxide is washed from their bloodstream. The patient complains of pins and needles in the hands and arms and the fingers and hands may be in characteristic spasm (Fig. 3.7). The feet may also be involved in carpopedal spasm.

Chronic respiratory conditions

In many cases these conditions will already have been diagnosed. The patient, friends and family will probably be experts. However, these patients can also suffer from other conditons which must be distinguished.

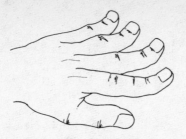

Fig. 3.7   Carpopedal spasm.

All of these patients will show signs of hypoxia and will be frightened and exhausted by their condition. Hypoxic drive may be present with any of these conditions. Pursed lip breathing may be evident.

Asthma.   This often occurs in a younger age group. Smooth muscle of the bronchioles goes into spasm, which, coupled with a production of mucus, allows the patient to inhale easily. Exhalation is both difficult and noisy. The presence of an inhaler is a good clue (see p. 86).

Chronic bronchitis.   Irritation of the bronchioles and the production of mucus reduces the useful area of the lungs. The patient is frequently cyanosed and shows signs of cardiac failure. A sensation of tightness in the chest may be reported.

Emphysema.   Bronchioles and alveoli are damaged. In addition, the lungs lose elasticity. Although cyanosis may be present, the patient will normally be pink. Breathing will be difficult, frequently in puffs through pursed lips.

Cardiac conditions
Cardiac arrest.   Signs of cardiac arrest are:

- Absence of the carotid pulse
- Cyanosis or ashen face
- Dilated pupils
- No respiration

ARRHYTHMIAS

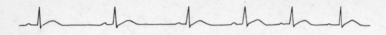

Fig. 3.8 Sinus arrhythmia.

Sinus arrhythmia (Rate = 60–100 beats/min regular rhythm).
There is irregular spacing of the PQRS complexes. An irregular discharge of impulses from the sinoatrial (SA) node causes alternating periods of slow and rapid rates. This is commonly associated with the phases of respiration. The faster rate occurs towards the end of inspiration and the corresponding period of slower rate occurs towards the end of expiration. This is due to reflex stimulation of the vagus nerve by receptors in the lungs. It is usually not found in patients over 30 years old.

Sinus arrhythmia is a common and harmless condition requiring no treatment. This condition is accentuated by digitalis and carotid sinus and eyeball compression, and is abolished by exercise and drugs such as atropine.

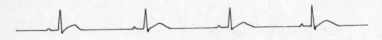

Fig. 3.9 Sinus bradycardia.

Sinus bradycardia (Rate = < 60 beats/min regular rhythm). This occurs when the SA node discharges at a rate of less than 60 beats/minute. It is a normal response to sleep. Athletes naturally develop a slow heart rate but compensate with a high stroke volume. It is also a reaction to raised intracranial pressure, obstructive jaundice and hypothyroidism. Sinus bradycardia is common following myocardial infarction as a result of vagal dominance over the SA node secondary to myocardial ischaemia and pain. It is also caused by drugs such as digitalis and beta-blockers.

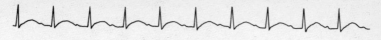

Fig. 3.10 Sinus tachycardia.

Sinus tachycardia (Rate = 100–130 beats/min regular rhythm).
This occurs when the SA node discharges at a rate faster than 100 beats/minute in adults. Reflects overactivity of the sympathetic nervous system in such conditions as anxiety, pain, physical exercise and hay fever. More importantly it arises as a sign of cardiac failure. The heart rate rises by reflex mechanism to compensate for reduced stroke volume. Can be induced by drugs such as adrenalin, dopamine, salbutamol, alcohol and by fever.

Heart block. This is a regular disturbance of rhythm. Conduction fails between the atria and the ventricles.
  Failure can be of three types:

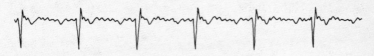

Fig. 3.11 Heart block—first degree.

1 First degree. The PR interval is extended but there is one P wave for each QRS.

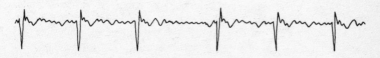

Fig. 3.12 Heart block—second degree.

2 Second degree.
  • Intermittent failure of conduction
  • Occasional P wave with no QRS
  • Cycle of lengthening PR interval and missed QRS
  • Ratio of P : QRS is 2 : 1 or 3 : 1

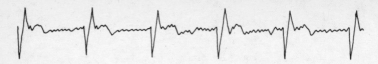

Fig. 3.13   Heart block—third degree.

3 Third degree. There is complete failure of conduction. P waves are not triggering QRS.

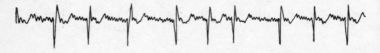

Fig. 3.14   Atrial fibrillation.

Atrial fibrillation. This is irregular rhythm, which may be slow or fast. Irritability of the atrial muscle causes irregular contraction which leads to irregular conduction to the ventricles.

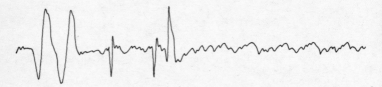

Fig. 3.15   Ventricular extrasystole.

Ventricular extrasystoles. These can occur with most heart rates. An irritable focus in the ventricles discharges prior to the next impulse from the SA node. There may be one or more foci giving rise to irregular extrasystoles. They are common following myocardial infarction and are likely to initiate ventricular tachycardia and ventricular fibrillation, especially when they occur R on T.

![Ventricular tachycardia ECG tracing]

Fig. 3.16 Ventricular tachycardia.

Ventricular tachycardia (Rate = 140–220 beats/min regular rhythm). Complexes are wide and regular. P waves are indefinable. Four or more consecutive premature ventricular contractions occur at a rapid rate. It can occur spontaneously but is more often due to myocardial irritability, especially following myocardial infarction. An ectopic focus within the ventricles sets the heart rate. It is often the prelude to ventricular fibrillation. Digoxin toxicity may suppress atrial activity, allowing a ventricular focus to take over. It may occur as a result of drug overdose, especially tricyclic antidepressants.

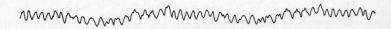

Fig. 3.17 Ventricular fibrillation.

Ventricular fibrillation (Rate > 140 beats/min).
The rhythm is rapid and irregular, with no definable complexes—electrical anarchy. **It is not detectable by pulse or heart sound**.

Electrical impulses arising in the ventricles repeatedly stimulate the muscles at a rate too fast to allow recovery. Muscle fibres are unable to fully contract but merely twitch.

It commonly occurs following myocardial infarction, frequently heralded by extrasystolic beats and/or ventricular tachycardia. Electrocution is also a common cause.

Myocardial infarction. Part of one of the coronary arteries is narrowed or occluded by atheroma or a blood clot. This leads to ischaemia or necrosis of the myocardium supplied by that vessel.

It can occur at rest, often some time after exertion, and is not completely resolved by rest.

The major symptom is pain in the chest, mostly in the sternal region, but it may spread to both sides of the chest, jaw, abdomen, shoulders and either or both arms. The patient describes the pain as pressing, tight, heavy or constricting. He may report a feeling of impending death. Remember the coronary is the great mimicker. The pain is often thought to be indigestion.

The patient is distressed, breathless, sweaty and cold. The pulse may be normal in rate and volume. In severe attacks it may be thready and fast. Blood pressure falls progressively over a period of hours or days. Hypertension is sometimes seen due to pain; otherwise, severe hypotension and cardiogenic shock may result. Nausea and vomiting are common. Arrhythmias appear in most patients with myocardial infarction during the first two hours. Infarction can exceptionally be painless, the so-called silent coronary.

Angina pectoris.   The coronary arteries, although not blocked, are narrowed and unable to supply the oxygen needs of the myocardium. Pain is brought on by exercise or emotion. The pain is retrosternal, often radiating to the neck, jaw and down the arm. Pain in the chest is often described as pressing, and in the arm as tingling.

Most attacks last only 1–3 minutes and seldom more than 15 minutes. If the patient has glyceryl trinitrite tablets the symptoms will be quickly relieved after one is placed under the tongue.

There are now sprays and gels for oral administraton of drugs to angina patients as well as pads for cutaneous absorption.

The first attack of angina pectoris should always be assumed to be a myocardial infarction until proved otherwise.

Heart failure.   The myocardium of the ventricles ceases to function normally. Left ventricular failure causes breathlessness because blood is not being drained from the lungs. This normally follows previous heart disease. The patient can be described as blue, breathless and bubbly.

Congestive heart failure is the failure of the right ventricle. Blood backs up in the venous system. Oedema is present with fluid gathering at the lowest point.

Shock

Shock is a series of signs and symptoms brought about by a reduction of effective blood flow around the body.

Signs and symptoms.   These are as follows:

- History of injury or disease
- Increased pulse rate
- Lowered blood pressure

- Cold, clammy skin
- Pallor
- Rapid, shallow respiration
- Vomiting
- Thirst

The decreased tissue perfusion can be seen in the lack of colour in the nail beds and the shut-down of the peripheral veins.

Causes of shock. These are as follows:

- Cardiogenic shock—diminished output of the heart
- Hypovolaemic shock—haemorrhage (internal or external)
- Metabolic shock—loss of fluids and changes in the body chemistry
- Respiratory shock—insufficient oxygen in the blood
- Neurogenic shock—loss of vascular system nervous control
- Psychogenic shock—reaction to certain stimuli
- Septic shock—toxins in the blood during severe infection
- Anaphylactic shock—acute allergic reaction to a foreign substance

Wounds

A wound is any disruption of the tissues. Wounds are classified by their cause:

- Contusion—a blow causes bleeding in the tissues
- Laceration—a torn, ragged, open wound
- Incision—clean cut; the wound may gape
- Puncture—a small skin wound with tissue damage related to the depth of the wound and the instrument
- Gunshot—a puncture wound with metal, clothing and skin often carried along the track. There may be an exit wound as well, characteristically larger than the entry wound, especially with a high velocity missile
- Degloving—skin is stripped off a limb
- Gravel rash—many small lacerations with contamination

Blood loss

Open blood loss can be seen, although it is necessary to check all over the skin of a patient. Open blood loss from, for instance, the back can soak into thick clothing.

Concealed blood loss is blood that gathers in a space within the body. This may be in the tissues following a broken limb, or in one of the body cavities. In limbs, concealed blood loss will cause some swelling (Fig. 3.18). When blood is lost into a body cavity, despite its large quantity, it may be undetectable for some hours.

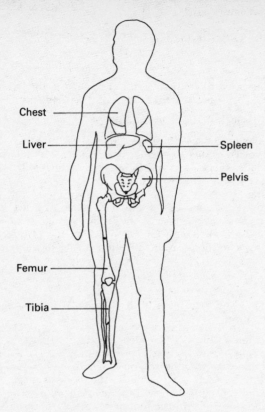

Fig. 3.18   Sites of concealed blood loss.

Estimation of blood loss.   To assess a patient's condition and the need for fluid replacement it is necessary to estimate the amount of blood lost (Fig. 3.19).

Tissue damage can be assessed by estimating the number of times that the patient's hand will fit over the wound. For deep wounds the fist is used. Each hand or fist is equivalent to 10% of the blood volume.

The total loss is the sum of the external blood loss plus the tissue damage.

- **10% blood loss** results in little or no sign of shock.
- **20% blood loss** results in an increased pulse rate, normal blood pressure and warm, pink extremities.
- **30% blood loss** results in an increased pulse rate and cold, grey extremities. Blood pressure may still be normal.

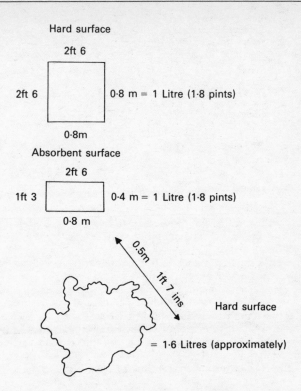

Fig. 3.19 The estimation of blood loss.

- **Above 30% blood loss** may result in very rapid changes.

In babies and children the small total blood volume must be taken into account when calculating the percentage blood loss. Children have circulatory systems that compensate well for blood loss. However, continuing blood loss will eventually cause an all the more sudden collapse.

Ruptured internal organs such as the liver or spleen may clot over whilst blood pressure is reduced by shock. Later, as blood pressure rises, these clots will give way suddenly.

TREATMENT

Resuscitation

Resuscitation is attempting to return the impaired physiology of the body to normal levels. There is a great variety of conditions,

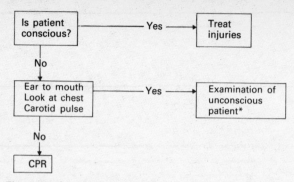

Fig. 3.20   Resuscitation—initial assessment. *See pp. 86–94.

both medical and traumatic, where resuscitation is required. Figure 3.20 shows the initial assessment and the immediate actions that follow.

Of overriding importance is the maintenance of a clear airway and the transport of oxygen to the tissues. There are a variety of procedures to facilitate this. Figure 3.21 shows how these procedures are put together for cardiac arrest. In all cases, where required, basic resuscitation must be commenced as soon as possible and continued without interruption. Resuscitation is about teamwork. The crew must be practised at switching from one to two rescuers during resuscitation. This allows further procedures to be carried out without interruption of the flow of oxygenated blood.

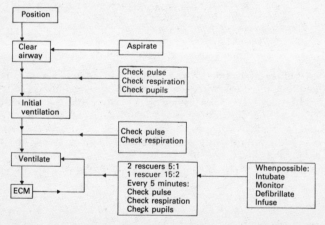

3.21   Cardiac arrest flow chart.

Positioning.   The following points should be noted:

- In order to maintain a patent airway, correct positioning is essential.
- If the patient is unconscious, but breathing spontaneously, insert a Guedel airway and place in the recovery position (Fig. 3.22). A close watch must be kept for any change.
- If cardiopulmonary resuscitation is to be performed, place the patient flat on his back. Tilt his head back with the atlas on the axis. Ensure a clear airway by holding the angle of the mandible forward. Failure to open the airway will allow air to enter the stomach, causing regurgitation of contents.

Obstruction.   The following steps should be taken:

- Remove the obstruction and create a clear, effective airway.
- Remove the foreign body with the fingers. Use a laryngoscope to see the object clearly. If the airway is still obstructed, give a sharp blow between the shoulder blades if practicable.
- Perform a Heimlich manoeuvre (Fig. 3.23). This works best when the lungs are full of air. Beware of causing injury and be ready to remove the foreign body.
- After clearing the airway, cardiopulmonary resuscitation may be required. If the patient is breathing but unconscious, insert a Guedel airway.
- Administer 50% oxygen.

Aspiration.   The obstruction may be regurgitated stomach contents, blood or inflow of foreign matter, e.g. teeth or peanuts.

Prompt removal of the obstruction is essential. Consider using a suction booster to augment the normal aspirator.

- Immediate treatment: commence aspiration with the patient on his side or with his head turned to one side. Then position the patient head down for optimal drainage.
- Ensure that no residual fluid remains by performing suction. **Beware of retching and further vomiting**. Maintain a head-down tilt.

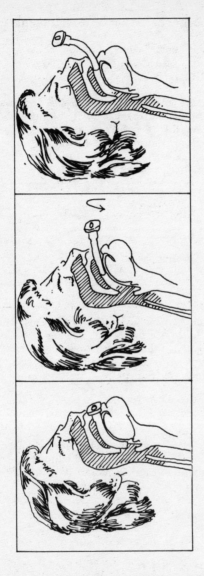

Sizes

4   Large adult
3   Adult
2   Small adult
1   Child
0   Baby
00 Small baby

Fig. 3.22 Insertion of a Guedel airway.

- Remove any false teeth. Beware of part plates that may slip into the pharynx. Ensure a patent airway using a Guedel airway and the recovery position or endotracheal intubation.

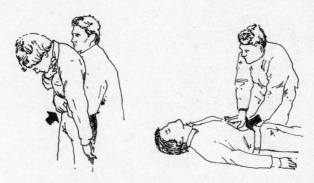

Fig. 3.23 Heimlich manoeuvre.

Commonly absent in other than specialist vehicles is a comprehensive selection of suction catheters. The recommended minimum is as follows:

- Flexible suction catheters in sizes 4–8 (infants) and 10–14 (adults)
- Rigid suction mounts
- Paediatric and adult disposable Yankauer

Suction, if performed properly, should not cause trauma and should be as aseptic as possible. A suction catheter should be connected to the aspirator and the tube occluded or vented for insertion. Suction is only applied during extraction. Keep the tube patent by sucking water through it between use.

Intubation.   Indications for intubation are as follows:

- To safeguard the airway in an unconscious patient
- Acute laryngeal obstruction
- Restoration of failed respiration

Intubation falls into two main categories: oral and nasal.

In an emergency, start with a Guedel airway bag and mask or a Brook airway. If difficult to intubate DON'T PERSIST, but go back to the technique that worked.

Even in ideal circumstances intubation may not always be possible. It is easier on a trolley stretcher than the floor if circumstances permit the transfer.

Intubation under direct vision of a trapped patient is only possible if access is possible above the patient's head. In an emergency, blind nasal intubation can be attempted as a last resort.

Equipment required

- laryngoscope
- selection of endotracheal tubes in the following sizes:

	Size (mm)	Cut length (cm)
Adult male	10.0	26
	9.5	25
Adult female	9.0	24
	8.5	23
14 years	8.0	22
12 years	7.5	21
10 years	7.0	20
8 years	6.5	20
6 years	6.0	19
4 years	5.5	17
2 years	5.0	15
1 year	4.5	14
6 months	3.5	12
Newborn	2.5	11

- Lubricating jelly
- 20 ml syringe
- Artery forceps (Spencer Wells)
- Bag resuscitator
- Suction unit comprising suction catheters and mounts and an optional suction booster
- Corrugated catheter mount and 15 mm connector

The procedure (Fig. 3.24)

> - Pre-gel the tube, particularly around the cuff.
> - Check that the cuff inflates and holds the pressure.
> - Reassure the patient; he may be aware of what is happening.
> - Check for and remove false teeth, and loose crowns if possible.

- Ideally, have the patient lying on his back with a Guedel airway in place.
- Use a bag and mask with 100% oxygen, and with the head fully extended.
- Stand or kneel behind the patient's head. Decrease the extension of the neck until the airway is straight.
- With all equipment to hand, pick up the laryngoscope with the left hand.
- Cricoid pressure is applied by the assistant in case of vomiting.
- Introduce the blade into the right side of the mouth and aspirate any secretions.
- Aim the laryngoscope blade for the mid-larynx without touching the lips or teeth. Follow the landmarks—the roof of the mouth, the uvula and the epiglottis.
- Lift, don't lever, the handle forward and upwards.
- The blade tip will rest just in front of the epiglottis, lifting it forward to give a clear view of the larynx. The vocal cords will now be visible.
- Insert an endotracheal tube down the right side of the mouth, through the glottis and just past the vocal cords. If there is any difficulty use a smaller tube.
- Once the tube is inserted, inflate the cuff.
- Connect a bag resuscitator to the catheter mount and commence inflation.
- Observe the chest for equilateral inflation. Listen to the apices with a stethoscope for air entry. If the right side only inflates, the tube may be in the right main bronchus. Let the cuff down and withdraw the tube 3–4 cm. Reinflate the cuff and try again.
- When the tube is correctly positioned, tie it in place and continue ventilation.
- Test for lung compliance with shallow respirations first. Do not overinflate.

If the patient gags or his cords close, STOP immediately.

Complications

- Obstruction of the tube with mucous plugs and secretions
- Kinking of the tube
- Leaking cuff
- Misplacement of the tube—too high or too low or in the oesophagus
- Pneumothorax from overinflation
- Vomiting
- Equipment failure

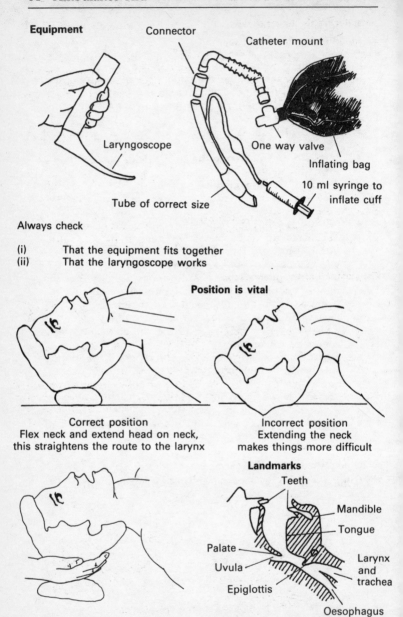

Equipment

Connector

Catheter mount

Laryngoscope

Tube of correct size

One way valve

Inflating bag

10 ml syringe to inflate cuff

Always check

(i)   That the equipment fits together
(ii)   That the laryngoscope works

Position is vital

Correct position
Flex neck and extend head on neck,
this straightens the route to the larynx

Incorrect position
Extending the neck
makes things more difficult

Landmarks

Teeth

Mandible

Tongue

Palate

Uvula

Epiglottis

Larynx and trachea

Oesophagus

The epiglottis covers the larynx

Fig. 3.24 Intubation.

Introducing the laryngoscope

Hold laryngoscope in <u>left</u> hand

Introduce the laryngoscope to the right hand side of mouth, deflecting the tongue to the left and aiming for the midline at the level of the larynx.

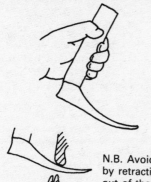

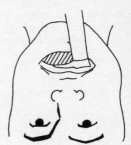

N.B. Avoid lower lip by retracting it out of the way

The position of the laryngoscope

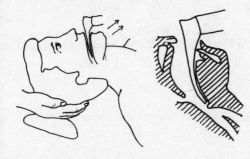

Insert tip of laryngoscope blade in groove between epiglottis and tongue to lift the epiglottis out of the way and expose the larynx

Draw larynx into line with mouth by upward and forward lifting of laryngoscope in line with the handle

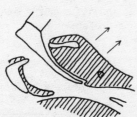

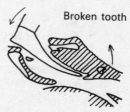

Broken tooth

Lift in this direction

This direction breaks off the front teeth

Ventilation.   There are three methods that ambulance personnel use to ventilate patients:

- Exhaled air resuscitation (EAR)
- Bag and mask
- Mechanical ventilators

All ambulance personnel are trained in EAR. This may be assisted by use of various types of intubation apparatus and masks. When using a mask, ensure that there is a good seal. Practice is the best way to perfect the technique (Fig. 3.25).

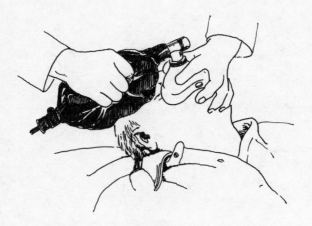

Fig. 3.25 Use of a self-inflating bag and mask.

When performed in conjunction with cardiac massage, inflations should be accomplished rapidly without interrupting compressions.

Whenever possible, 100% oxygen should be used for resuscitation.

Initially, four quick inflations are given, not allowing full exhalation. This helps to open up the collapsed alveoli.

Check for adequate ventilation by:

- Seeing the chest rise and fall
- Feeling the lung compliance (only with EAR and bag and mask)
- Hearing and feeling the air escape with each exhalation

The lungs should be inflated 12 times/minute for adults, 15 times/minute for children of 1–8 years old, and 20 times/minute for children under 1 year old. The pressure and volume used for children must be reduced to avoid lung damage. Use either an infant resuscitator or EAR, using the cheeks, not the diaphragm.

Crews must be fully conversant with their equipment, which they must have checked.

If it is necessary to move an intubated patient, one connector should be left relatively loose. Should anything catch, the connection will then break. Reconnection is easier than reintubation.

Oxygen therapy.   The purpose of oxygen therapy is to optimize the supply of oxygen to the tissues and reduce the load on the respiratory and circulatory systems.

The factors affecting oxygen concentration in the tissues are:

- The oxygen concentration in the inspired gases
- The minute volume (volume of inspiration multiplied by the number per minute)
- The state of the circulatory transport system

1 *Oxygen concentration.* This is determined by the flow rate and mode of delivery. For resuscitation using a ventilator or bag and mask with oxygen, the concentration will be up to 100%.

Where a disposable mask is used, the concentration at the mouth is set by the flow rate (Fig. 3.26). Masks which allow rebreathing cannot be guaranteed to supply a particular concentration at low minute volumes.

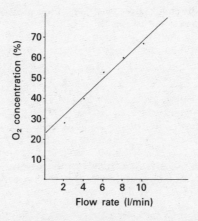

Fig. 3.26   Oxygen concentration against flow rate, using a typical disposable oxygen mask.

As a basic rule trauma and sudden illness require a high concentration (50%) and chronic respiratory conditions require a slightly raised concentration (30%).

2 *Minute volume*. Oxygen shuttled up and down the dead space will not benefit the patient. Respiration must be deep enough to change the gases in the alveoli. If necessary, in an unconscious patient, respirations can be deepened with a bag and mask. Inspirations should be timed to coincide with the patient's efforts.

3 *The state of the circulatory transport system*. Oxygen must be transported from the alveoli to the tissues. To do this the circulation must have sufficient volume and pressure. Increasing the concentration will overcome slight transport insufficiency. Further steps that should be taken are the positioning of the patient and the correction of any arrhythmias.

Gases such as carbon monoxide reduce the ability of blood to absorb oxygen. Treatment consists of increasing the oxygen concentration after removing the source. Maximum use is made of unaffected haemoglobin.

Problems of oxygen therapy

Fire risk of oxygen means that ignition sources and oil or grease must not be allowed near patients receiving oxygen therapy. This applies both inside an ambulance and outside in a wrecked car or a factory.

Entonox, containing 50% oxygen, also poses a fire risk. A rise of 5% oxygen concentration in a confined space will quadruple the explosion hazard. Always inform firemen when oxygen is in use.

Patients in hypoxic drive may respond to oxygen therapy by respiratory arrest. It is for this reason that chronic respiratory patients should not receive high oxygen concentrations. Treatment consists of immediate resuscitation using normal air.

External chest compression (ECC) (Fig. 3.27)

- The patient must be on a hard surface.
- The patient's body must be flat. If the legs can be raised without delay, this is an advantage.
- Hands must be positioned over the lower third of the sternum, not overlapping onto the ribs. In children the heart is positioned higher in the chest. So:

     For infants, two fingers should be placed on the mid-sternum.

     For children, one hand should be placed 1 cm higher than on adults.

- The rescuer's arms should be kept straight, with the

force provided by a transfer of weight through a rocking movement.

● Each compression should take 1 second, with equal time spent at the bottom and top of the compression cycle.

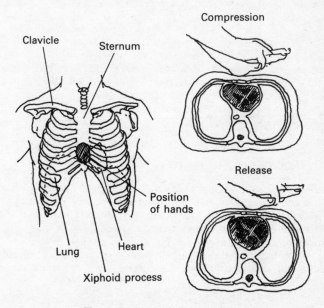

Fig. 3.27 External chest massage.

Defibrillation. When the heart is in ventricular fibrillation whether coarse or fine, the electrical impulses are 'firing' (depolarizing) in individual muscle fibres out of synchrony. The heart is reduced to an unpalpable quiver with no measurable cardiac output. This condition can only be accurately diagnosed by electrocardiogram. However, if no device is available and all signs indicate cardiac arrest, assume ventricular fibrillation and treat accordingly.

In the event of ventricular tachycardia the rapidity of persistent contractions may give rise to a low systolic blood pressure (<60 mmHg).

The ultimate aim in either case is to resynchronize the electrical activity of the cardiac muscle fibres. To do this a large number of fibres must be made to contract at the same instant. The heart will then hopefully restart 'in step'. The earlier that defibrillation is carried out following ventricular fibrillation, the greater the chance of recovery. However, the myocardium must be well oxygenated. Good cardiopulmonary resuscitation must be started before defibrillation is commenced.

A defibrillator is a capacitor for stored electrical energy, measured in joules, and delivers an impulse of direct current.

Procedure

The operator must be fully conversant and practised with the equipment before usage. All models have the same main function controls:

- An on/off switch
- A joule rating selector
- Defibrillator paddles with discharge buttons

Once switched on, the desired joule rating is set. The unit will take a few seconds to charge. **DANGER: THE UNIT IS NOW POTENTIALLY LETHAL**.

A good electrical contact is made between the patient and the paddles by using a conducting gel and firm pressure. These measures not only ensure a good contact but also prevent scorching of the patient's skin.

Saline-based gel should be applied to both paddles in sufficient quantity to coat the surface. The gelled paddles should be applied at the contact points (Fig. 3.28).

The operator should ensure that:

- They are not kneeling in water, urine or any other liquid
- No-one is in contact with the patient
- The patient is not in contact with conducting objects
- No jelly bridges the gap between the paddles
- The clear, audible warning 'Stand Clear' is given and a visual check is made before pressing the discharge buttons

There is much debate about the energy required. As a rule the larger the patient the higher the energy needed.
Adults
First shock: 200 J
Second shock: 200 J
Third shock: 400 J
Fourth and subsequent shocks: 400 J

Children
10–12 years: 100 J
5–9 years: 50 J

2–4 years: 25 J
0–1 year: 10 J

In the absence of paediatric defibrillator paddles, a child can be laid on its side. Defibrillation takes place from front to back (Fig. 3.29).

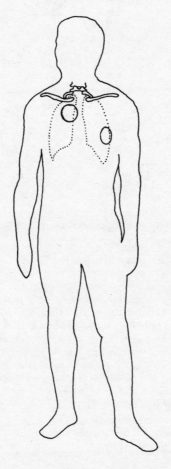

Fig. 3.28   Defibrillation—position of paddles.

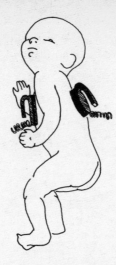

Fig. 3.29 Defibrillation of infants using adult paddles.

Safety

Defibrillators can be as deadly as they are life-saving. They should only ever be used by personnel trained to use them.

Equipment, especially paddles, must be kept clean and dry. Jelly smeared up the handles is a potential source of danger. Cracked or broken paddles or connections must be replaced.

Ambulance personnel may be called upon to use equipment in hostile environments. The golden rule is if you are not happy, then don't use it. If it is raining, consider moving the patient to the ambulance whilst continuing cardiopulmonary resuscitation. If this is not possible, get somebody to shelter you. Dry the skin between the paddles. If your hands are wet, even surgical gloves will protect you.

Defibrillators must not be used in an explosive atmosphere. Drugs are sometimes administered via pads in contact with the skin of the abdomen. These must be removed before defibrillation or explosion may result.

Infusion

Indications for cannulation

- To give access to a vein soon after or during trauma
- To facilitate fluid replacement/resuscitation
- To allow the bolus injection of drugs

Contraindications

- Heart failure (extra volume would increase the load on the heart)
- Head injury without shock from other trauma
- If attempted cannulation fails, don't waste time and sites.

Sites of choice. In an emergency any vein that is palpable may be used, although it is best to steer clear of sites over joints.

If there is a choice of veins the larger one closest to the trunk is the best. When no other vein is available the external jugular vein can be used.

Equipment
- Cannula
  Sizes
  Extra large, 14 g, brown, for rapid infusion
  Large, 16 g, grey, for rapid infusion
  Medium, 18 g, green, for general use
  Small, 20 g, pink, for children
- Alcohol wipes
- Securing tape
- Infusion fluid
- Giving set

Method of cannulation

- The giving set should be connected to the infusion fluid (Fig. 3.30).
- Reassure the patient and explain what you are going to do (see chapter 1).
- Either get an assistant to manually squeeze the limb or use a constricting band. The venous return is occluded and the veins become engorged.
- Palpate and stabilize the selected vein. Stretch the skin away from the intended site of puncture.
- Clean the skin at least 2 cm around the puncture site.
- Introduce the needle through the skin, then advance into the vein either from the side or above.
- Insert the cannula for 1–2 cm, withdraw the needle 2–3 cm, and advance the cannula 2–3 cm.
- Withdraw the needle totally. Apply finger pressure over the vein to prevent bleeding.
- Use an obturator to seal the entry port unless infusion is to commence immediately.
- Tape the cannula in place. Splint the limb if required. Use anchor strapping to fix the tube high up the arm. This reduces the risk of pulling on the cannula.

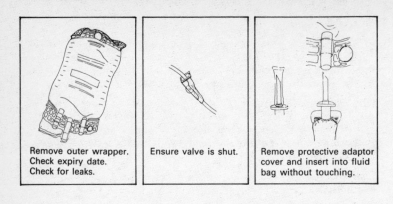

Remove outer wrapper.
Check expiry date.
Check for leaks.

Ensure valve is shut.

Remove protective adaptor
cover and insert into fluid
bag without touching.

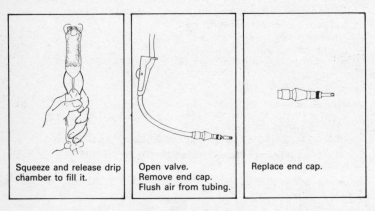

Squeeze and release drip
chamber to fill it.

Open valve.
Remove end cap.
Flush air from tubing.

Replace end cap.

Fig. 3.30 Connecting a giving set.

Transport

Shocked patients need to arrive in hospital as soon as possible
after treatment has been given. However, a rough ride will dislodge
clots that have formed. A patient who has survived an accident
will become unduly anxious if the ride is not smooth.

Resuscitation in the back of a moving ambulance is not easy. If
arrest occurs during transport, the driver should stop and assist
until the patient is stabilized. The ride can be fast in a straight
line on a smooth surface, but care must be taken on bends that
the attendant does not lose his balance.

Cardiac cases require gentle transport. The use of audible
warning systems is normally not beneficial. Care should be taken

when starting up or down steep hills or turning sharp corners. Cardiac arrest can be triggered by acceleration forces and bumps.

Use and care of equipment

Equipment for cardiopulmonary resuscitation is the most important carried on an ambulance. It must be, at all times, complete, in the correct place and guaranteed to work, with spares at the ready.

Each person has their own preferences for the details of their own equipment. Only a few important points are included here:

Masks.   Different sizes of mask are required; 0.2 and 5 are usual. Check them regularly for splits and keep them clean.

Resuscitators.   All push-fit parts are better when they are put together with a quarter turn. They stick better and will not come apart so easily. Check that valves are clean and that they work. Check especially that exhalation is possible. Any person using a resuscitator must know the procedure for clearing vomit from the valves.

Defibrillators.   Care must be taken that the paddles are clean. This prevents current tracking to the operator, pitting of the paddles and subsequent burning of the patient.

Cardiac monitors.   Patient electrodes are notoriously difficult to peel and fix when in a hurry. Keep them attached, ready for use.

Suction equipment.   A selection of catheters should be available and their sizes should be readily identifiable. Manufacturers could help by improving the packaging.

Wounds

The aim of treatment is:

- To arrest haemorrhage
- To promote clotting
- To prevent the entry of infection

The stages in dealing with wounds are as follows:

- Apply direct pressure over the wound with a clean dressing.
- Reassure the patient.
- Elevate the affected part if practical.
- Be ready to apply further dressings over the top if blood soaks through the dressing.
- Treat shock if present, and monitor and record the vital signs.
- Transport the patient smoothly to his treatment.

There are further considerations which may apply to certain wounds: Blood is an alkali. It reacts with clothing materials and dyes. Wherever possible, clothing should be cleared from around a wound at an early stage.

Loose foreign material, especially if sharp, should be removed before applying a dressing if blood loss is not rapid.

Impaled objects must be left in place. Great damage may be done by movement or withdrawal. A ring pad should be used to provide support of the protruding part. Occasionally it will be necessary to cut objects, such as railings, before the patient can be removed. The assistance of the fire brigade will be required. This task must be undertaken methodically, bearing in mind the following:

- At least 10 cm of the object should be left protruding.
- Cutting produces heat. Heatban putty, copper wire or running water will prevent this affecting the patient.
- The patient and the object must be supported during cutting.

Occasionally, direct pressure will not stop haemorrhage. In other instances impaled objects prevent its use. Figure 3.31 shows pressure points. The use of pressure points is as an adjunct to other means of stopping haemorrhage and their use should not be prolonged.

Specific conditions

Cardiac conditions. The overall aim of treatment is to relieve pain and reduce the load on the heart. Reassurance is essential.

Conscious patients should be carried in a semi-recumbent position. Unconscious patients should be laid flat in the recovery position unless intubated.

Monitor electrodes should be applied before commencing the journey so that changes in condition can be recorded. Remember that the most common imitator of asystole is a detached lead.

Pain can be relieved by use of Entonox (p. 132). In addition, this gives 50% oxygen. If pain is not great 50% oxygen should be given to patients who appear hypoxic.

Angina patients who have medication with them should be encouraged to take their normal dose. Vital signs and arrhythmias should be recorded. This information must be handed over to the medical staff at the hospital. In particular, details of ventricular extrasystoles will determine the priorities for the medical staff.

Shock. This should be treated thus:

- Maintain an adequate airway. Administer oxygen ensuring a good minute volume.
- Control any bleeding. Gain access to a vein and infuse if appropriate.
- Reassure the patient and give pain relief.

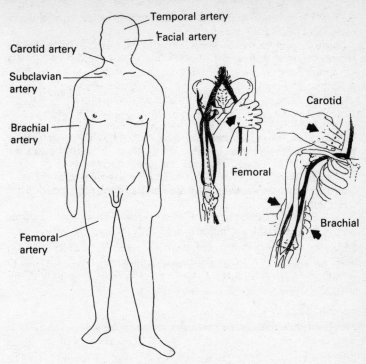

Fig. 3.31 Pressure points.

- Position correctly. Keep the patient lying down. Apply a head-down tilt if injuries permit.
- Give nothing by mouth; lips can be moistened.
- Prevent loss of body heat but guard against overheating. Feel the patient's forehead since they may shiver even when hot.
- Transport to hospital without delay but avoid rough handling.

Drowning.   Whether drowning is wet or dry the treatment is the same. Ventilation should commence as soon as possible, ideally in the water. Oxygen enrichment during resuscitation is useful. Maintain a head-down tilt; the stomach may be full of water, which may be regurgitated. Look for and treat arrhythmias, especially ventricular fibrillation. Prevent loss of body heat but do not rewarm: sudden opening up of the peripheral circulation will withdraw blood from essential organs. Especially if a patient is found in cold water, do not give up attempts at cardiopulmonary resuscitation. Time limits for brain death may not apply if the body is kept cold.

In cases of near drowning where the patient has been unconscious, removal to hospital is essential. Secondary drowning may set in later.

Smoke inhalation. Treatment consists of resuscitation as required followed by oxygen therapy. Transport to hospital is always necessary as bronchitis and pneumonitis may develop later.

Asthma. Reassurance, support and encouraging the patient to use his inhaler are all of benefit. In addition, the condition of the patient must be closely observed for any deterioration.

The use of oxygen-powered nebulizers to administer bronchodilator drugs such as Ventolin (salbutamol) has done much to improve treatment.

The nebulizer can be used either with the vehicle oxygen supply or with a portable supply. Patients must be relaxed before treatment. To do this they should be:

- Supported in an upright position with pillows reaching up to and including the head
- Told to remain motionless and calm
- Reassured and their anxiety allayed

Some patients are hot and will benefit from cool air.

At this stage the nebulizer is assembled and the nebule squeezed into the container. The oxygen supply is set at 4 l per minute. The mask is then put on the patient.

The patient is encouraged to relax and reminded that his difficulty is an inability to breathe out. After three or four breaths through the mouth and a deep breath out, he is encouraged to take a deep breath in. Then the patient is told to relax and breathe normally.

An occasional deep breath in, preceded by a long breath out, will ensure that the Ventolin pervades as much of the lungs as possible. Ventolin only acts on the lung tissue, and if the patient remains tense the effect of the drug can be negated. When the solution has been totally nebulized, the mask is gently removed and the patient kept relaxed for as long as possible—a minimum of 20 minutes.

In addition, the following points are important:

- The attendant must be calm and reassuring.
- The patient's chest should be massaged one side at a time to coincide with breathing out, in order to assist exhalation.
- A small adhesive label is affixed to the patient stating that he has been nebulized and the date and time.

Patients must be relaxed and supported. They must not be left alone and the treatment must not be interrupted.

Hysterical hyperventilation.   The aim of treatment is to restore a normal pattern of breathing. This is achieved by getting the patient's confidence, slowing the rate and lessening the depth of breathing, and increasing the carbon dioxide in the blood.

Reassurance and firm instructions are needed. If pain is the cause of the hyperventilation, steps should be taken to relieve it.

In the absence of chest injury, firm pressure on the ribs with the hands, allowing the patient to breathe at a normal rate, will often achieve a good result in 2 minutes.

Another method of restoring a normal pattern of breathing is to get the patient to breathe into a paper bag. This works well but requires considerable confidence on the part of the patient.

4

The Nervous and Sensory Systems

The activity of the nervous system can be observed by assessing the presence or absence of activity in systems under its control. The special senses and other systems of the body provide a window on the nervous system. To interpret the information it is necessary to understand the working of the system and how it exercises its control.

ANATOMY

The central nervous system

The central nervous system comprises the brain and spinal cord. Contained within the meninges, it is bathed in cerebrospinal fluid (CSF).

The brain. The brain fits tightly inside the skull, following the contours of the bone. Figure 4.1 shows the principal parts, external areas and functions of the brain. The blood supply to the brain is shown in Figure 4.2. The blood is isolated from the brain tissue by the capillary walls. Venous blood collects in sinuses and returns to the heart via the internal jugular and vertebral veins.

When intracranial pressure is raised there is little space for expansion. Consequently, brain tissue is compressed. Pressure on the reticular activating system alters the level of consciousness, and excessive pressure can force the medulla oblongata down through the foramen magnum. This is termed 'coning'.

Meninges. The central nervous system is surrounded by three membranes—the meninges. The pia mater follows the contours of the brain and contains very fine capillaries. The arachnoid contains a large number of blood vessels. It dips between the major convolutions of the brain and contains the CSF within it. The dura mater is in two parts: the outer forms the periosteum of the skull and the inner serves to contain the brain.

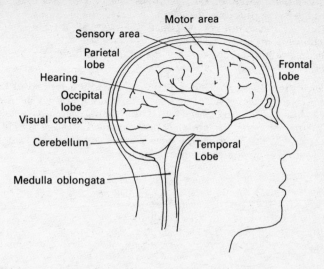

Fig. 4.1 The principle parts, external areas and functions of the brain.

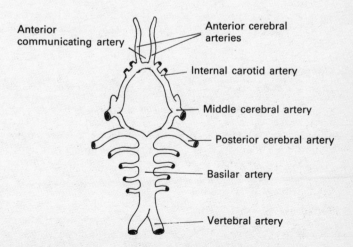

Fig. 4.2 The blood supply to the brain—the circle of Willis.

Any inflammation of the meninges leads to pressure on the nerves passing through the skull, such as the auditory nerve. Rupture of the meninges potentially allows CSF to escape and infection to enter.

The meninges, except the pia mater, extend down the spinal column further than the spinal cord.

Cerebrospinal fluid.   CSF is a straw-coloured fluid formed in the choroid plexus. Figure 4.3 shows the arrangement of the ventricles of the brain. CSF circulates around the central nervous system, maintained at a pressure normally in the region of 60–150 mmH$_2$O.

Fracture of the surrounding bones and meninges can lead to CSF issuing from the ears, nose or mouth.

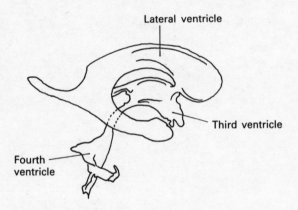

Fig. 4.3   The arrangement of the ventricles of the brain.

The peripheral nervous system

There are three components of the peripheral nervous system:

- Cranial nerves—issuing from or terminating directly in the brain
- Spinal nerves—arising from or terminating in the spinal cord
- Autonomic nervous system—linked to the spinal cord indirectly by a series of ganglia and to the tenth cranial nerve (the vagus)

Cranial nerves.   See Table 3.

Spinal nerves.   See Figure 4.4.

Autonomic nervous system.   This is made up of the sympathetic and parasympathetic nerves that control involuntary muscles and

Table 3. The cranial nerves.

Cranial nerve	Type	Function and distribution
1 Olfactory nerve	Sensory	The nerve of smell. Starts in the nose and passes to the olfactory bulb.
2 Optic nerve	Sensory	The nerve of sight. Starts in the retina and passes to the lateral geniculate body.
3 Oculomotor nerve	Motor	Arises in the mid-brain and ends in the muscles which move the eye.
4 Trochlear nerve	Motor	As for the third cranial nerve.
5 Trigeminal nerve	Motor and sensory	Supplies the muscles of mastication. Sensory nerves branch from the face.
6 Abducent nerve	Motor	Arises in the pons and ends in one of the muscles moving the eye.
7 Facial nerve	Motor and sensory	Supplies the muscles of facial expression. Sensory nerves arise from the tongue.
8 Vestibulocochlear nerve	Sensory	The nerve of hearing and sense of balance.
9 Glossopharyngeal nerve	Motor and sensory	The nerve of taste. Motor fibres lead to the pharynx.
10 Vagus nerve	Motor and sensory	Supplies the heart and the digestive tract, controlling both secretion and movement.
11 Accessory nerve	Motor	Supplies muscles of the neck, pharynx and soft palate. •
12 Hypoglossal nerve	Motor	Supplies the tongue.

glandular secretions. There is no conscious control over these nerves.

Oedema of nervous tissue

If ventilation is impaired the PCO_2 rises and the PO_2 falls. Both of these factors cause vasodilatation, so the amount of blood inside the skull increases. Such raised intracranial pressure depresses the medulla oblongata, containing the respiratory centre, down into the foramen magnum. Respiration is depressed, completing the vicious circle. Figure 4.5 shows the cycle which, if uninterrupted, leads to death.

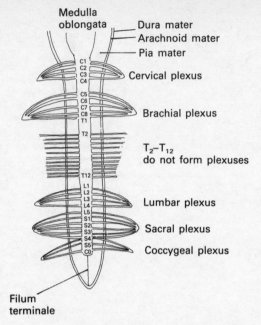

Fig. 4.4 Spinal nerves and plexuses.

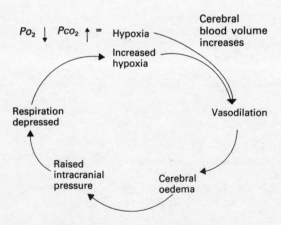

Fig. 4.5 The effect of hypoxia on the brain.

The spinal cord is also contained in a limited space. Bruising causes oedema, increased pressure and further damage.

The special senses

Sight, hearing, smell and taste make up the special senses. Sight is of particular importance in diagnosis for the information it reflects of the activity of the brain.

Figure 4.6 shows the arrangement of the visual pathways. The third cranial nerve—the oculomotor nerve—controls the pupil reaction. When functioning normally, light shone in one eye stimulates both sides of the visual cortex. Feedback via the oculomotor nerve causes both pupils to constrict. This is termed 'the consensual light reflex'.

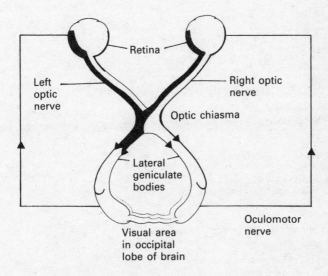

Fig. 4.6   The arrangement of the visual pathways.

Damage to an area of the brain involved in this process or pressure on the oculomotor nerve can cause deviation from the norm.

Causes of unconsciousness

Unconsciousness is a loss of awareness. This is brought about by pressure or chemical deviation acting on the reticular activating system (RAS). The major causes of unconsciousness are:

Brain disease or injury

- Head injury
- Cerebrovascular accident
- Infection
- Cerebral tumours
- Cerebral oedema
- Epilepsy

Cardiorespiratory disease

- Hypovolaemia
- Hypoxia
- Carbon dioxide retention

Drugs and toxins

- Alcohol
- Tranquillizers
- Carbon monoxide
- Hepatic
- Uraemic coma

Endocrine disorders

- Diabetes
- Myxoedema
- Steroid shock

Electrolyte disorders

- Dehydration
- Sodium depletion
- Potassium depletion

Temperature disorders

- Hyperthermia
- Hypothermia

DIAGNOSIS

Examination of the unconscious patient

A patient with an impaired level of consciousness is at risk as he cannot look after himself. Therefore it is necessary to carry out an assessment, to care for the patient while at the same time arriving at a diagnosis. Figure 4.7 shows the sequence of steps.

Approach. The patient is unconscious for a reason. Ambulance personnel must make sure that they do not succumb to the same

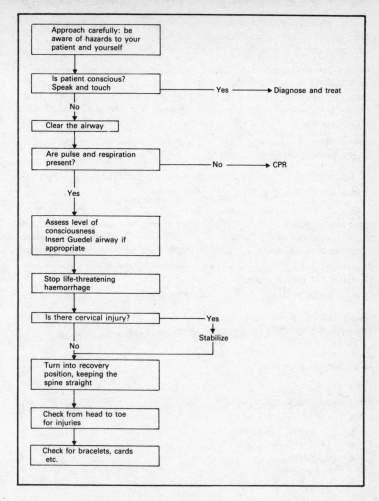

Fig. 4.7 Examination of the unconscious patient.

cause. Look for, and ask bystanders about, the history. Toxic gases, electric current and falling objects are all risks that may prevent immediate access to the patient.

Do not make assumptions. Presence outside a bar smelling of alcohol is not conclusive evidence of intoxication.

History taking may continue throughout the examination. A patient who has been unconscious will not be a reliable provider of information. What the patient can supply is the length of time before and after the accident during which he had amnesia. This has considerable relevance to the severity of injury.

Initial assessment. As soon as the patient can be safely approached, an initial assessment is made. This assessment is the same as that in chapter 3. The nature and rates of pulse and respiration should also be noted. Assess the patients overall. Do they look shocked? Do they feel cold?

Level of consciousness. There are two reasons for noting the level of consciousness:

- To monitor any change in the patient's condition
- To assess the level of risk to the airway

Tests used must be capable of being repeated by others to obtain equivalent assessments. There are scoring systems, such as the Glasgow coma scale, which should be used where ambulance services and hospitals have specifically agreed a common system.

Glasgow coma scale.
The scale is divided into three sections:

Eye opening
- Spontaneous
- To speech
- To pain
- Not at all

Best motor response
- Obeys commands
- Localizes pain
- Withdraws from pain
- Extensor response
- No response

Best verbal response
- Orientated
- Confused conversation
- Inappropriate words
- Incomprehensible sounds
- None

Eye opening is not, on its own, a good indicator of the level of consciousness. To apply pain, pinch the trapezius muscle at the base of the neck. This can be done out of sight of bystanders.

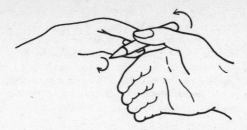

Fig. 4.8 Applying a painful stimulus.

Motor responses on both sides of the body should be tested. When a patient localizes pain he uses a limb in a positive attempt to remove the stimulus. The painful stimulus to use is the side of a pen rolled over a nail bed (Fig. 4.8).

When assessing verbal response be aware that some patients may not have appeared to be orientated before the accident.

If the cough reflex is absent then the patient will accept a Guedel airway (see chapter 3).

Life-threatening haemorrhage. Only bleeding from a major vessel need be controlled at this stage. Blood soaking into clothing and inside boots is hard to see and must not be ignored.

Cervical injury. Forces sufficient to cause head injury are potentially able to cause cervical injury. Feel gently for irregularity of the cervical spine. If in any doubt or if the history is uncertain, stabilize with a cervical collar and appropriate lifting.

Recovery position. Turning the patient into the recovery position may need to be done at any stage if the patient appears to be about to vomit. *A clear airway takes precedence over all other measures.*

The patient's spine should be kept straight whilst turning so as not to aggravate any spinal injury (Fig. 4.9).

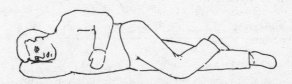

Fig. 4.9 The recovery position adapted to keep the spine straight.

Check from head to toe. A detailed examination of the patient may have to wait until the patient is loaded into an ambulance. Heavy clothing will hinder diagnosis and extremes of cold and wet will not benefit the patient. A balance must be struck erring on the side of caution.

All possible sites of bleeding must be checked. Keep looking at your hands to see if blood has appeared on them. Check for puncture wounds and discoloration of the skin, which may indicate internal bleeding.

Carefully check for fractures remembering that the patient may not respond to pain. Crepitus should always be treated as a definite indication of fracture. Avoid causing further damage.

Note any movements that the patient makes. Has he moved all his limbs? Paralysis of a limb is hard to diagnose in an unconscious patient. In the absence of spontaneous movement, differences in muscle tone give some indication.

Diagnostic evidence. Even with a full history from bystanders, written evidence will aid diagnosis. This may be in the form of a necklace, bracelet or card giving medical information. Alternatively, there may be indirect evidence such as sugar lumps or appointment cards.

In addition to aiding diagnosis, a name and address is useful information for the hospital. Take care to explain to bystanders that you are going to examine a patient's property, and do not hide what you remove. If a policeman is present ask him to take charge of all property not required by the hospital.

Pupil reactions. Of great importance in the hand-over report is a clear record of pupil reactions and changes. Depending on the length of journey and the workload it may not be possible to check pupil reactions more than once, but this still provides valuable information.

The information is most easily recorded on a patient report form. These vary from service to service (Fig. 4.10). The information required is:
- Time of examination
- Approximate size of pupil (can be marked on a scale)
- Speed of reaction (normal/sluggish/absent)
- Consensual light reflex (present/absent)

Each pupil reaction must be recorded separately so that there is no confusion between the left and right pupils.

Head and maxillofacial injury

Injury to the brain can be caused by direct force, acceleration and deceleration forces, or indirect force transmitted up the spine. There are several distinct types of injury:

Patient Report Form

INJURY ASSESSMENT/PRIORITY	
Critical/Immediate	☐
Serious/Urgent	☐
Moderate/Delayed	☐
Minor	☐

Crew	Dr.	Nurse	
Date		Call Time	
Location		Arrival Time	
		Depart Time	
Hospital		Arrival Time	

Surname   Forename   M/F

d.o.b.   Address

TYPE OF INCIDENT RTA ☐ Home ☐ Works ☐ Organised Sport ☐ Leisure ☐ Other (Specify) ☐

If RTA: Driver ☐ Front/Rear Passenger ☐ Pedestrian ☐ Motor-cyclist ☐ Cyclist ☐

Seatbelts? Yes ☐ No ☐ Not known ☐ Vomited? Yes ☐ No ☐ Alcohol? Yes ☐ No ☐ Not known ☐

Crash helmet? Yes ☐ No ☐ Not known ☐ Ko'd Yes ☐ No ☐ Trapped? Yes ☐ No ☐ How long?

OBSERVATIONS	Time	1)	2)	3)
Appearance	Pallid	☐	☐	☐
	Cyanosed	☐	☐	☐
Blood Loss	Slight	☐	☐	☐
	Moderate	☐	☐	☐
	Severe	☐	☐	☐
Blood Pressure		—‐—	—‐—	—‐—
Pulse Rate				
Respiratory: Rate				
CNS Eye Opening	Fitting	☐	☐	☐
	Spontaneous	4 ☐	☐	☐
	To voice	3 ☐	☐	☐
	To pain	2 ☐	☐	☐
	Nil	1 ☐	☐	☐
Best Verbal Response	Orientated	5 ☐	☐	☐
	Confused	4 ☐	☐	☐
	Inappropriate	3 ☐	☐	☐
	Incomprehensible	2 ☐	☐	☐
	Nil	1 ☐	☐	☐
Motor Response	Obeys command	6 ☐	☐	☐
	Localises pain	5 ☐	☐	☐
	Withdrawal (pain)	4 ☐	☐	☐
	Flexion (pain)	3 ☐	☐	☐
	Extension (pain)	2 ☐	☐	☐
	Nil	1 ☐	☐	☐
Pupils	React R	☐	☐	☐
	(√ or X) L	☐	☐	☐

1 ○ Constricted   Size R
2 ○ Normal
3 ○ Dilated   L

INJURIES

C#	Closed Fracture
O#	Open Fracture
B	Burn (shade area)
F.	Foreign body
L	Laceration
A	Abrasion

Bowel Sounds
☐ Present
☐ Absent

ACTION TAKEN		Dose/Volume	Time
IV Fluids	☐ N. Saline		
	☐ Hartmans		
	☐ Haemaccel		
Other (specify)	☐		
Analgesia/ Drugs (specify)	☐ Entonox		
	☐		
	☐		
Cardiac Arrest	☐ ECM		
	☐ Defib.		
Airway	☐ Airway ☐ Oxygen ☐ Sucker		
	☐ Ventilated ☐ Intubated ☐ Mini Trac		
Splints	☐ Cx Collar ☐ Hines ☐ Box		
	☐ Frac Straps ☐ Inflatable ☐ Traction		

COMMENTS:

Signed Crew	Dr.	Nurse

HOSPITAL FOLLOW UP	Hospital No.
Diagnosis A/E	A/E No.
Disposal	DOA ☐ ADM ☐ OP ☐ Home ☐
Died Date	Time
Trauma Score Time 1)	2) 3)

© Copyright C.J. Eaton 1987

Fig. 4.10 An example of a patient report form.

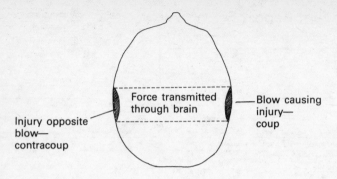

Fig. 4.11 Coup and contracoup injuries.

Concussion. This is manifested by a disruption of mental activity following a blow to the head. Signs and symptoms vary considerably with the severity of the blow. Concussion is often present in addition to other conditions. Signs and symptoms are:

- History of a blow to the head
- Evidence of loss of consciousness
- Mental confusion
- Amnesia
- Nausea
- Pulse rapid and feeble
- Skin pale, cold and clammy
- Breathing low and shallow
- Pupils equal
- Severe headache
- Blurred vision

Contusion. This occurs as a result of force transmitted through the skull, causing bruising to the brain. Injury may be coup or contracoup (Fig. 4.11).

Signs and symptoms are initially similar to concussion. Later, pupil and limb reactions may become unequal. There may be cerebral irritation with the patient being very restless and vomiting.

Laceration. This consists of damage to brain tissue caused by bone fragments and/or foreign objects entering the skull.

Signs and symptoms are similar to those found in contusion. In addition it may be possible to find the depressed fracture or entry point. Where the possibility of a depressed fracture exists, the skull must be felt carefully to search for a boggy mass under the scalp.

Compression. Raised intracranial pressure commonly follows serious brain injury, especially if ventilation is impaired. Occasionally it may be caused by bleeding from the middle meningeal artery. A small quantity of extruded blood will fill all the available space within the skull. This amount of bleeding does not produce signs of shock. Compression may not occur for several hours.

Signs and symptoms are:

- History of a head injury
- Lucid interval after a period of unconsciousness
- Face becomes flushed
- Pusle slow and full
- Blood pressure raised
- Body temperature raised
- Breathing stertorous
- Pupils unequal
- Convulsions

Lucid interval

Compression most often develops in a patient who is or has been suffering from concussion. As the brain recovers from concussion the level of consciousness rises. If compression develops the level of consciousness will diminish. A lucid interval is a period of consciousness in between the two conditions which is revealed by the accurate recording of the conscious level. This provides an accurate diagnosis of compression. Figure 4.12 shows the possible outcome of head injuries.

Fractures of the skull

These may complicate head injury in the following ways:

- Fragments may lacerate the brain.
- Displacement may damage nerves or brain tissue.
- Infection and contamination may take place.

Depressed fractures may be felt by gentle pressure. Other signs of fracture are blood and/or CSF issuing from the ears, nose or mouth. Fractures of the front of the base of skull produce vivid bruising around the eyes confined to the orbital area.

Cerebrovascular accident (CVA)

This is caused by an embolus, thrombus or haemorrhage in the cerebral circulation and is most common in elderly hypertensive individuals.

Signs and symptoms vary a great deal and may develop and subside in the course of a few hours or days. Some of the following may be present:

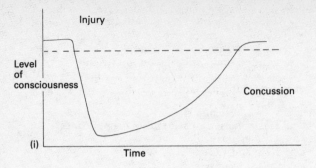

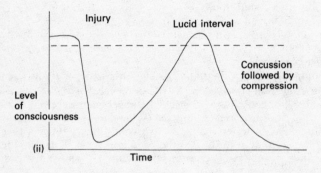

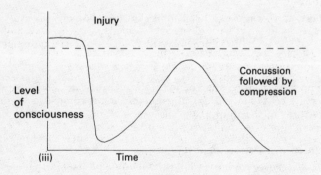

Fig. 4.12 Levels of consciousness. (i) Patient unconscious after injury gradually regains consciousness. (ii) Following concussion compression causes a second loss of consciousness. (iii) Compression intervenes before patient regains consciousness.

- Sudden onset preceded by headache
- Unconsciousness
- Confusion, if conscious
- Pulse full and rapid
- Breathing difficult and noisy
- Collapse due to loss of limb function
- Paralysis or weakness of one or more limbs
- Distorted facial expression
- Pupils unequal
- Eyes looking to one side
- Speech impaired or absent
- Nausea and vomiting

Inflammation of the nervous system

There are a wide number of infective conditions that affect the nervous system. Those that cause inflammation of the meninges are termed 'meningitis'. Inflammation of the meninges can also be caused by the presence of blood in the meninges, as in subarachnoid haemorrhage.

Inflammation of the brain itself is termed 'encephalitis'. In the pre-hospital phase it is hard to distinguish the type of infection. Signs and symptoms of nervous system infection are:

- Headache
- Fever
- Confusion
- Photophobia (dislike of light)
- Neck rigidity and pain on flexion or extension

Epilepsy

There are two types of epilepsy—generalized and focal. In both types the fits may vary in severity. Epilepsy may occur at any age. It may occur following neurosurgery or due to a brain tumour, but usually the cause is unknown.

Generalized epilepsy. This can be petit mal with only a momentary loss of consciousness, such as a pause in conversation. This is most common in children. Grand mal is the recognizable fit which follows definite stages:

- Aura or prodrome—the patient may experience a feeling which he recognizes as a warning.
- Tonic stage—the muscles contract violently for a period of 30 seconds to a minute. Cyanosis occurs as a result of respiratory muscle spasm.
- Clonic stage—violent alternate flexor and extensor muscle contractions, frothing at the mouth and snapping of the jaw, lasting for 2–3 minutes.
- Resting—the muscles relax and the patient appears to be asleep. The patient may be incontinent. Consciousness gradually returns but the patient is amnesic of the event.

Status epilepticus. Occasionally one fit follows another with only a short pause. This is extremely exhausting for the patient. Without drugs, fits may continue until death.

Focal epilepsy. Symptoms vary greatly but are generally not as severe as a grand mal fit. Typically there is an aura stage followed by violent or uncharacteristic behaviour of which the patient has no knowledge or recollection.

Spinal cord injury

It is possible to sustain damage to the bony structures of the spine without damage to the spinal cord and vice versa. After a fall the patient may be lying with the spine in the normal posture. The history may suggest that during the accident extreme flexion or extension took place.

The signs and symptoms of spinal injury are dealt with in chapter 2. The level at which cord damage takes place determines the signs and symptoms:

- **Upper cervical injuries** cause paralysis of breathing and remove the feedback control on the heart.
- **Injuries at the level of the fifth cervical vertebra** cause paralysis of all breathing muscles except the diaphragm and paralysis of both arms and legs.
- **Thoracic and lumbar injuries** may result in an uneven paralysis of muscle groups. They are sometimes associated with the patient lying with the hands up (Fig. 4.13). The upper limbs may escape paralysis. Loss of bladder control may lead to acute retention.

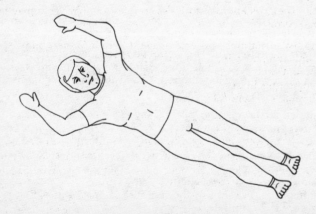

Fig. 4.13 Uneven paralysis of muscle groups may lead to the patient lying in the hands-up position.

Cord damage may only be due to bruising, causing a tingling feeling in the limbs. However, this may be followed by further oedema of the cord, giving rise to further symptoms and deterioration. Following spinal cord injury the blood pressure may fall because of disruption of the autonomic feedback control. In any recently injured patient this cause of reduced blood pressure must not be accepted until blood loss can be ruled out.

Peripheral nerve injury

The peripheral nervous system can be damaged wherever a nerve is squeezed against a bone. In many cases the damage is slight and recovery is complete. However, more serious damage can cause permanent disability. The injury may result from:

- Direct trauma—a cut or a blow damaging the nerve
- Pressure—seen especially in unconscious patients with limbs hanging over the side of a trolley or with tight splints or bandages.
- Stretching—holding the patient by the limbs

Early signs of pressure on a nerve are:

- Pain
- Pins and needles
- Anaesthesia
- Paralysis

Unconscious patients and those with spinal cord injury are especially prone to peripheral nerve damage because they are unable to complain of pain.

Injury to special senses

Eyes. The eyes are the most susceptible to injury. This may take several forms:

- Corneal irritations and/or damage due to a foreign body
- Blunt trauma—a blow compressing the eye in the orbit
- Foreign body—irritating or abrading the cornea
- Penetrating injury
- Thermal or chemical burns

Corneal irritation and damage
Diagnosis is made from the patient feeling the foreign body in the eye. Careful note should be made of the history. The velocity of the foreign body is important. High velocity dust, for instance from a grinding wheel, may have penetrated the eye, whereas dust blown into the eye will be easily removed.

Blunt trauma
This is caused by a blow from an object that is small enough to compress the eye without bearing on the bones of the face. The

eyelids will often have closed before contact, but this does not rule out disruption of the internal structures. Swelling may well prevent examination of the eye. However, if examination is possible, careful note should be made of abnormalities since swelling may take place later.

The eye is a delicate structure. During exposure to heat the lids will usually close, protecting the eyes. However, sudden heat, such as after an explosion, may burn the corneal surface. Damage from chemicals is more severe from alkalis than from acids. Relatively weak solutions will cause severe pain.

Penetrating injury
Sharp objects such as tree branches or darts may penetrate the eye. If the object is no longer in the eye, diagnosis is made from the history and the visible wound. The pupil may become irregular.

Ears. The pinnae bleed profusely if they are cut or torn. Bleeding from within the ear is usually due to a fracture of the base of skull. CSF may be visible, mixed with the blood.

After exposure to excessively loud noise, especially explosions, the patient may become deaf or complain of ringing in the ears (tinnitus).

Inflammation of the ear may cause intense pain and nausea and interferes with balance.

Nose. The bones of the nose are often fractured as a result of their prominent position. This is accompanied by bleeding— epistaxis. This must be distinguished from bleeding resulting from head injury and fracture of the base of skull.

TREATMENT

Patients, especially those with a reduced level of consciousness, must be protected from further harm. Reassurance is important. Because a patient does not respond does not mean he is not aware. Hearing is often the last sense to lapse, the patient reporting conversations after recovering consciousness.

Head injury

It is not possible to treat brain damage caused by injury. It, is, however, possible to minimize the damage caused by hypoxia and cerebral oedema subsequent to injury.

The principles of treatment are to:
- Clear and maintain the airway and good ventilation
- Ensure adequate oxygenation of the tissues
- Protect the patient from further injury
- Record the vital signs and the level of consciousness at timed intervals
- Transport the patient to hospital
- Hand over the patient, giving all relevant information

Airway

Methods of clearing the airway are dealt with in chapter 3. If there is any suspicion that there might be injury to the cervical spine, then the neck should not be flexed, extended or rotated.

To maintain a clear airway positioning is of great importance. The recovery position (Fig. 4.9) with a Guedel airway, if the patient will accept it, is the preferred method. The patient must not be left alone.

A trapped patient who is unconscious is at great risk. Intubation to safeguard the airway may be possible if the level of unconsciousness is sufficiently deep. Otherwise all efforts must be directed at basic methods of airway control while releasing the casualty sufficiently to allow him to be turned.

Oxygenation of the tissues

A clear airway in itself is not enough. Ventilation and circulation must be sufficient to oxygenate the tissues and prevent cerebral oedema (Fig. 4.5).

Oxygen should be given to patients suffering from head injury. The depth and rate of breathing must be monitored. If the minute volume starts to decrease, breathing should be assisted using a bag and mask with oxygen enrichment, timed to coincide with the patient's breathing to enhance each breath.

Loosen tight clothing around the neck to encourage venous return from the head and neck.

Head injury does not produce shock. It may, however, be present due to other injuries. Where shock is present with head injury then the source of bleeding must be found.

Where head injuries are associated with maxillofacial injuries, use of an oxygen mask is not acceptable. Oxygen can be administered using high flow rates via an open tube close to the mouth.

Recording vital signs

Decisions regarding the management of a patient in hospital may be taken as a direct result of information gathered by ambulance personnel. It may not be realistic to carry out observations at set intervals; rather, the time of observation should be recorded. Ideally observations should be carried out on arrival at the scene and at not less than 15-minute intervals.

Transport

Patients with head injury should be turned in the recovery position. If intubated they may be laid on their back. A head-down tilt is contraindicated because it increases intracranial pressure.

Whenever the patient is touched or moved he should be informed what is happening whether he is conscious or not.

The head-injured patient urgently needs to be transferred to hospital. However the ride must be smooth enough to allow accurate observation of the patient. Noise levels should be kept low. Many unconscious patients become disturbed by the use of audible warning systems.

Hand-over

Information must be recorded in writing. At hand-over, ambulance personnel should ensure that medical staff can understand the written information.

Motor-cycle helmets

Immediate removal of the visor is necessary to prevent rebreathing. Removal of a helmet is a difficult procedure. If the patient is able to do it himself, this is preferable. If it causes no problems then it can remain in place. With full face helmets it is not possible to maintain a clear airway without removing the helmet. Figure 4.14 shows how this is accomplished.

Spinal cord injury

Lifting and transport of the patient with spinal injury is dealt with in chapter 2. The spinal cord is part of the central nervous system and suffers oedema in the same way.

High spinal cord injury may cause a fall in blood pressure. This must be distinguished from hypovolaemic shock, and intravenous fluids should not be administered in large amounts.

Low blood pressure leads to reduced peripheral circulation and the skin becomes vulnerable to pressure necrosis. It is not possible, under normal circumstances, to turn patients in an ambulance. Wrinkled bedding and pressure from side bars should be avoided.

Reassurance is of the utmost importance. Diagnosis of cord injury by the patient is not uncommon, causing great anxiety. Pain relief should be given once the patient is properly positioned.

Cerebrovascular accident

The principles of treatment are as for a head injury. Frequently the patient finds it difficult or impossible to speak. Ambulance personnel must find ways of communicating; touch is useful when combined with reassuring words. Eye movements or gripping with a good limb can provide a method of communication for the patient.

The conscious patient will be more comfortable in a semi-recumbent position. Vomiting is frequent following a cerebrovascular accident and the airway should be assumed to be at risk.

Myocardial ischaemia is often associated with cerebrovascular accident. Patients showing signs of a cardiac problem should be monitored accordingly (see chapter 3).

Release chin strap, open visor, remove spectacles, false teeth etc.

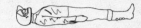

Prepare to turn into recovery position.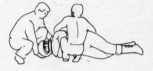

Place palm of hand inside helmet against patient's cheek. Steady head as patient is turned.

Keep patient's spine straight as he is turned.

Keeping hand on cheek, grasp chin piece and rotate helmet to clear jaw. Rear of helmet must not press on cervical region.

Ease helmet upwards and backwards to complete removal, ensuring head is supported at all times.

Fig. 4.14 Removing a full-face motorcycle helmet.

Infections of the nervous system

The risk of infection to ambulance personnel is small since the infection is well contained (see chapter 9).

The symptoms may cause the patient severe pain and he should be moved very carefully.

Bright light can be painful and ambulance blinds and eyepads help to alleviate this.

The patient's perception may be disturbed and quiet reassurance will be necessary. The ride should be smooth and quiet.

Epilepsy

Muscular action by the patient is extremely violent. Attempting to insert a gag in the mouth may do more damage than good. Of greater use is guiding the patient away from potential danger.

As soon as the clonic stage has finished, assist the patient into the recovery position. If the fit has occurred in the patient's home, transport may not be necessary if supervision is adequate. In a public place the patient will need to be transferred to hospital.

Some patients appear to recover quickly and get up soon after the fit. Such patients may be suffering post-epileptic automatism. They carry out actions without conscious decision and must be protected from harm. A firm order will usually be obeyed.

Peripheral nerve injury

Prevention is better than cure. Look for and remove pressure and allow the limbs to lie naturally. There are many potential ways of suffering peripheral nerve injury including:

- Wrist drop from a sling
- Arm hanging over the side of a stretcher
- Hitting the patient's elbow putting poles into a canvas
- Damage to peripheral nerves on the lateral side of the knee
- Temporary damage due to a 'bad' recovery position

Injury to the special senses

Eyes. It is important that the eyes of an unconscious patient should not be allowed to dry out or be damaged by dust or other foreign bodies. Dust and dirt will settle on the cornea. Gentle massage over the lids will often close them or they may be taped closed. Beware of tape loosened by tears touching the cornea.

Heat and chemical burns

Following heat and chemical injury the first essential is copious flushing. In factories handling chemicals there may be special solutions in containers for flushing eyes. If such solutions are not immediately to hand use clean water, provided that the chemicals are not water-reactive. This can be done either by the patient holding his face in the water and blinking, or by running a stream of water across the eye, moving the lids with the fingers.

Foreign bodies

Low velocity foreign bodies may be removed with a fine corner of cotton wool (Fig. 4.15).

High velocity foreign bodies may be stuck to the cornea where they have embedded. They are best left, the eye closed, covered with a pad and the patient transported to hospital.

Ears. Bleeding from tears or cuts of the pinnae requires pressure to stop the bleeding. Bleeding from the ears as a result of skull fracture should be absorbed in a pad. The pad should be lightly taped in place, preferably with the injured side down. The purpose of the pad is to prevent infection.

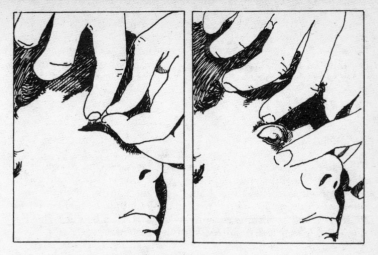

Fig. 4.15 Everting the eyelids.

Nose. Epistaxis should be treated by sitting the patient forward and getting him to pinch his nose just below the bony part. Pressure should be maintained for at least 5 minutes. If it does not stop in that time then pressure should be reapplied until arrival at hospital.

The patient should be encouraged to breathe through the mouth. Should bleeding stop then the patient must be reminded not to blow his nose and dislodge the clot.

Bleeding, especially in the elderly, may be torrential. It may be from the back of the nasal cavity and may not be stopped by simple pressure. Such patients may need to be treated for hypovolaemic shock. Care must also be taken of their airway.

Transport to hospital may need to be rapid but must not be rough.

5

The Digestive System

The digestive system is responsible for breaking down and absorbing the nutrients required by the body. Injury, although not common, is often serious. Both injury and non-injury conditions often produce severe pain. Treatment by ambulance personnel is limited. Good reporting can aid medical staff and much can be done to alleviate pain and reassure the patient.

ANATOMY

Regions of the abdomen

For the purposes of description the abdomen is divided into nine regions. Figure 5.1 shows the regions related to external landmarks and the organs within those regions.

It should be noted that the lower borders of the ribs overlap the abdomen, giving protection in part to the liver and spleen.

There can be considerable variation of position of the organs in the abdomen. The stomach and bladder, as they fill and empty, displace other organs. The bladder, for instance, rises out of the pelvis into the hypogastrium when distended.

Organs of digestion

See Figure 5.2.

Peritoneum

The peritoneum is a serous membrane in two layers: the parietal layer, which lines the abdomen, and the visceral layer, which covers the organs. The peritoneum does not line the whole abdomen. The organs are surrounded to varying degrees by folds of the membrane. There is a considerable amount of space to allow fluid to gather with little external sign.

Blood supply

All the digestive organs require large blood supplies to carry absorption products, to fuel muscle activity, and, in the case of the liver, to distribute heat as well.

104

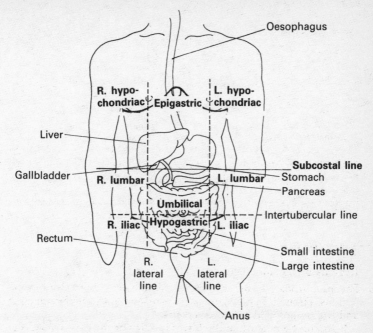

Fig. 5.1 Regions of the abdomen.

The most common site of bleeding is from the stomach, duodenum and oesophageal varices. Injury can affect the liver or spleen, both of which may bleed profusely. Delayed bleeding may occur where clotting gives way as blood pressure, reduced by shock, rises, or where the clot is disturbed or absorbed.

Nerve supply

Many of the abdominal viscera change position during development of the fetus. The sensation of pain is felt where the organs were positioned during development, at a distance to their true location. The common example is the pain of acute appendicitis which is first felt in the umbilical region. Likewise, pain in the shoulder may be referred from below the diaphragm.

Branches of the same nerves supply the peritoneum and the muscles of the abdominal wall. Thus peritonitis—irritation of the peritoneum—causes the muscles to tense and produce guarding. The viscera are not well supplied with sensory nerves. The peritoneum is very sensitive and is responsible for the majority of pain felt after injury or inflammation.

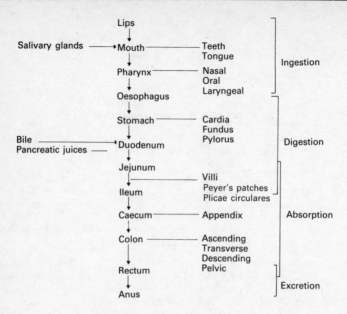

Fig. 5.2 The organs of digestion.

Muscles of the abdomen

The abdominal wall is made up of several layers of muscle. These lie at an angle to one another. The muscle of the diaphragm closes the abdomen from the thorax with communication for the oesophagus and major vessels. The muscles of the pelvic floor in part support the viscera.

The iliac and psoas muscles run obliquely against the peritoneum. These large muscles push against the abdominal contents when flexed.

DIAGNOSIS

In the conscious patient a history of pain is usually the major symptom.

In addition, vomiting may have taken place. Normal vomit consists of partly digested food. If the patient has not eaten for some hours, mucus and clear fluid may be all that is brought up. Where vomiting occurs repeatedly it is usual for bile to be brought up. This may be yellow or green. Blood in vomit may be fresh red or in dark clots. More often it is described as looking like coffee grounds; this is altered blood.

Blood may be present in the stools. Fresh blood is usually from haemorrhoids. Malaena—digested blood from higher up the digestive tract—presents as black, shiny, tarry stools with a characteristic odour.

Bowel sounds are hurried after injury, then become quiet before finally ceasing.

The history of the injury may seem trivial. Quite small forces can produce serious injury. Careful examination may be needed to find the injury, especially with penetrating wounds.

The presence and age of operation scars should be noted. The patient can often provide information based on previous knowledge. Previous operations may be associated with adhesions and partial obstruction of the intestine.

In women of child-bearing age, pregnancy is a cause of abdominal pain that must be considered. Similarly, the pain of myocardial infarction can be felt in the abdomen.

Examination of the abdomen

The patient must be reassured and as relaxed as possible before and during the examination. Attend to disorders of airway, respiration and circulation before commencing.

Examination proceeds in a logical order:

- Take the history whilst assessing the general condition, pulse and blood pressure.
- Remove clothing, if privacy is possible, and look for bruising on the abdominal wall.
- Are there signs of guarding (the abdomen held rigid, not moving with respiration)?
- Slide warm hands over the abdomen, feeling for guarding. Feel in each of the four quarters of the abdomen.
- Press more firmly over the abdomen, watching the patient for signs of tenderness.
- If tenderness is found, press again on the tightened muscles to determine whether the pain is superficial or deep.
- A sudden release of pressure on the abdomen sometimes produces pain. This is rebound tenderness caused by irritation of the peritoneum.
- Listen with a stethoscope for bowel sounds.
- Measure the girth with a tape measure between pen marks so that measurement can be accurately repeated.

Types of pain

Asking about the type of pain is of use in diagnosis. There are two basic types of abdominal pain: colic and peritoneal pain.

Colic pain. The pain is sharp and can be pointed to. The severity rises and falls. The patient is restless and moves about.

Peritoneal pain. The patient lies still, the legs drawn up. Pain is constant and aggravated by any movement or pressure.

Injury conditions

Injury conditions can be divided into 4 classes:

- **Bruising** caused by a fall or blow may be very painful but recovery commences in a few minutes. Shock is not present.
- **Rupture** of an organ will produce shock although, exceptionally, this may be delayed for up to several days. Usually there will be bruising over the site. The most common organs ruptured are the liver, spleen and large intestine.
- **Puncture**. Unless the cause is left sticking in the abdomen, the wound may be insignificant in appearance or hard to find. The internal situation may be very different, depending on the depth of penetration.
- **Prolapse**. The abdominal contents protrude through a natural or artificial orifice. Commonly following large abdominal wounds, the bowel protrudes through the wound. The protruding contents may be ruptured as well.

Non-injury conditions

Ambulance staff will be asked to deal with a great variety of non-injury conditions. Exact diagnosis is not possible or necessary. What is needed is the recognition of peritonitis and blood loss. Accurate reporting of signs and symptoms will help eventual diagnosis in hospital.

Signs and symptoms of peritonitis are:

- Severe pain which is continuous and made worse by movement
- Tenderness and rebound tenderness
- Guarding
- Raised temperature
- Rapid pulse
- Absent bowel sounds

Blood loss can be diagnosed by observing:

- Signs of shock (see chapter 3)
- Haematemesis and/or malaena
- Signs and symptoms of peritonitis

TREATMENT

Injury conditions

In the minutes following an accident it is not possible to positively diagnose that an injury is solely bruising. Rupture of an organ with delayed bleeding must always be considered a possibility.

A patient with an injury to the abdomen will require:

- Reassurance and pain relief
- Treatment for shock
- Careful lifting so as not to disturb the abdominal contents (remember that the lower ribs or pelvis may also be involved)
- A smooth ride that will not disturb blood clots
- Hand-over of all details at the hospital

Wounds

Wounds of the abdomen do not bleed excessively unless the viscera are themselves damaged.

Puncturing objects should not be removed. Dressing should be packed around the object to check bleeding and support the object. Should the object have been removed prior to arrival of the ambulance, a firm dressing is all that is required.

Prolapsed viscera should not be replaced. They need to be kept warm, moist and clean. The whole area should be irrigated with normal saline fluid, e.g. from a drip set, then covered with a large, clean dressing.

Non-injury conditions

Treatment follows the same lines as for injury conditions. Vomiting may require the conscious patient to be sat up and turned to one side, or the unconscious patient to be placed in the recovery position.

Pain relief

Entonox (see p. 132) is effective. However, reassurance and positioning both assist pain relief. Supporting the drawn up knees—Fowler's position—relaxes muscles, relieving pressure on the viscera.

6

The Urogenital System

ANATOMY

The organs of the urinary system and reproduction are contained in the abdomen and pelvis. Figure 6.1 shows the organs of the urinary system. The urinary system is also important for its functions of controlling the metabolism.

Kidneys

The kidneys lie on either side of the body high in the posterior region of the abdomen behind the peritoneum and embedded in perirenal fat. They are partially protected by the eleventh and twelfth pairs of ribs. The right kidney is slightly lower than the left because of the area occupied by the liver. At the centre of the concave aspect of each kidney is the hilum through which the ureter, blood and lymphatic vessels communicate with the kidney. Three layers of tissue surround each kidney, forming a capsule.

Ureters

The ureters are the two tubes which convey urine from the kidneys to the bladder. Each is between 25 and 30 centimetres long and 3 millimetres wide. They run behind the peritoneum and in front of the psoas muscle. They enter the bladder obliquely so that when the bladder is full the ureters are closed.

Bladder

The bladder is a reservoir for urine. Shaped like an inverted pear the neck of the bladder is fixed behind the pubic symphysis. As the bladder fills, so the upper surface rises into the abdominal cavity. The urge to micturate is felt when about 250 millilitres of urine have collected in the bladder. However, the bladder can hold up to 500 millilitres, although this causes pain.

Urethra

In the male the dual function urethra is 18–20 centimetres long, while in the female it is only 4 centimetres long. The urethra lies

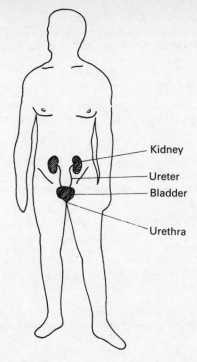

Fig. 6.1   The organs of the urinary system.

within the arch of the pubic bones. It can be injured by involvement in fracture of the pelvis as well as by direct trauma.

Function of the kidneys

The main task of the kidneys is as a regulator for the body fluids. This is accomplished by carefully balancing the composition, volume and pressure of the fluids. This balance is controlled by the rate of excretion of water solutes.

The critical biochemistry necessary for the whole body to function normally is controlled by the careful balance maintained by the kidneys. Overall control is by the pituitary body via hormones in the blood.

Fluid balance

The normal fluid requirement for a healthy individual is 2–3 litres/day. The majority of this is taken in through the digestive system. A small amount is formed by metabolic processes.

Water within the body is held within three fluid-containing compartments. These compartments are separated by semi-permeable membranes which permit the process of osmosis to take place.

Approximately 70% of the weight of the human body consists of water. This can be divided into:

- 50% contained within the body cells (intracellular fluid)
- 20% contained within the body fluids (extracellular fluid)

The extracellular fluid can be further divided into:

- 15% of body weight contained within the tissues (interstitial fluid)
- 5% of body weight contained within the blood, lymph and plasma

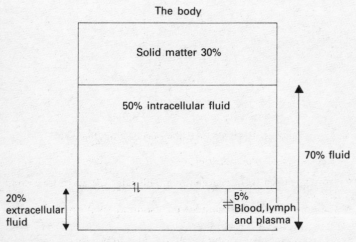

Fig. 6.2 Fluid-containing compartments within the body.

The average adult takes in approximately 2.5 litres of fluid per day, of which a similar volume is excreted via various routes (Fig. 6.3).

Electrolyte balance

The molecular content of the fluids must also be balanced if the body is to function normally. This is called 'electrolyte balance' and is achieved by the regulation of ions (electrically charged atoms or molecules).

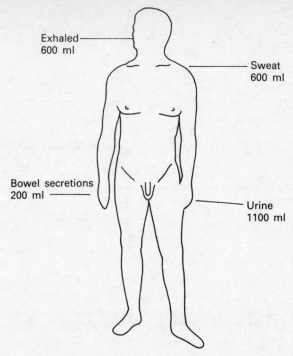

Fig. 6.3 The daily excretion of fluid from the body.

There are two types of ions:

- Anions—negatively charged, e.g. chloride (Cl) and bicarbonate (HCO_3)
- Cations—positively charged, e.g. sodium (Na) and potassium (K)

The totals of anions and cations determines the acid–base balance.

Acid–base balance

The acid–base balance of the body is maintained by controlling the hydrogen ion concentration of the body fluid, in particular the extracellular fluid. This is measured on a pH scale (Fig. 6.4).

The normal pH is maintained by buffers—the respiratory and renal function. The buffers include carbonic acid, bicarbonate, phosphate, haemoglobin, oxyhaemoglobin and protein.

- An increase in respiratory rate = a raised pH
- A decrease in respiratory rate = a lowered pH

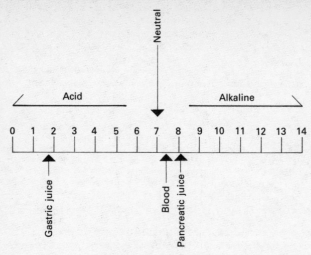

Fig. 6.4 The pH scale.

A blood pH between 7.35 and 6.80 is termed 'acidosis', the main effect of which is depression of the central nervous system.

A blood pH between 7.45 and 8.00 is termed 'alkalosis', the main effect of which is overexcitation of the central nervous system.

Respiratory acidosis is caused by hypoventilation and metabolic acidosis from an abnormal rise in acid metabolic products and loss of bicarbonate. This may occur, for instance, after cardiac arrest.

Respiratory alkalosis is caused by hyperventilation, and metabolic alkalosis results from non-respiratory loss of acid or excess intake of alkalis and/or drugs.

DIAGNOSIS

Trauma

Trauma to the genitourinary tract is generally characterized by either puncture or blunt injury. In severe cases it will be necessary to transport the patient to hospital as soon as possible in order to preserve the function and viability of the system.

Kidney. Kidney trauma may be caused by:

● Puncture—gunshot or stabbing

- Blunt injury—sports injuries, a fall or a punch. Often the twelfth rib can squeeze the kidney against the lumbar spine.
- Fracture of the lower ribs—subsequent injury may be puncture or blunt.

Signs and symptoms are:

- History of injury to the kidney
- Haematuria (not always present)
- Pallor
- Acute abdominal or loin pain
- Tachycardia
- Hypotension
- Bruising, haematoma
- Inability to micturate
- Palpable mass may rarely be felt at the location of the kidney

Physical examination may demonstrate a haematoma over the area of the eleventh or twelfth rib, indicating retroperitoneal haemorrhage.

The injuries that may have been sustained are:

- Contusion—may give rise to haematuria
- Laceration—may be capsular or pyramidal
- Rupture and/or fragmentation—may lead to urinary extravasation and disruption of the blood circulation

Ureters.   Direct injury to the ureters is relatively rare unless associated with penetrating injuries.

Diagnosis is made by noting a history of the injury in the appropriate area coupled with the diagnosis of haematuria and painful micturition. This would have to be confirmed by special investigations carried out in hospital.

Bladder.   Trauma to the bladder is rare. It may be injured by a fracture of the pelvis or by concussion against the symphysis pubis. A full bladder may be compressed by a seat belt in a high speed crash.

Rupture of the bladder usually occurs at its weakest point—the dome—and invariably when it is full. Empty bladders will not rupture.

The patient is usually unable to pass urine.

Urethra.   Trauma to the urethra will render the patient unable to pass urine. There may be blood present at the meatus in males, most easily noticed by looking at underclothing when the patient is undressed in hospital. By virtue of the longer urethra it is more prone to injury in males than in females.

Causes of injury to the urethra are:

- Blunt injury—direct blow, such as a kick in the crutch
- Shearing—a fracture of the pelvis
- Rupture—the insertion of foreign objects

The urethra is also often damaged in injuries to the perineum. This is commonly seen where motor-cyclists have gone forward onto prominent petrol caps at high speed.

Genitals. Injuries sustained by males are typically crush or laceration injuries. Injuries sustained by females tend to arise from penetrating or blunt trauma.

Examination of the genitals of a patient is not usually possible by ambulance personnel. The patient's modesty must be observed at all times. If the patient refuses to allow examination, this must be respected. Examination by someone of the same sex usually is less stressful to the patient. Under no circumstances should examination be undertaken without a witness being present. Ideally this should be an acceptable third party such as the husband or wife of the patient. Careful explanation and a professional manner are very helpful.

Miscellaneous injuries. The injuries in this category may be caused by:

- Sexual experimentation
- Sexual deviation
- Sexual encounter
- Self-inflicted wounds under the influence of drugs or alcohol
- General skylarking
- Other injuries as part of a sexual attack

Such injuries are embarrassing to the patient who may well not admit to being injured. Only a calm, non-judgemental attitude will prise out the necessary information.

Males

Any constriction around the penis causes swelling and pain. This may be from objects such as elastic bands or curtain rings. It may also be from an overtight foreskin—paraphymosis.

The erect penis, if bent excessively, may be reported as 'fractured'. This will be associated with pain and haematoma.

Objects may be passed into the urethra. These may rupture the wall of the urethra, effectively closing it off.

Females

Injuries are usually from the insertion of foreign objects. There is a severe risk of bleeding.

Young boys

In young boys a common occurrence is the 'bitten willy' syndrome where the penis is trapped in the zip fly following micturition.

Medical conditions

Various medical conditions affect the urinogenital system. Signs and symptoms may well present as an acute abdomen.

Renal calculi/colic. Stones formed in the kidneys—calculi——sometimes pass into the ureters. This can cause acute and severe pain. The patient may appear pale, sweaty and prone to vomiting.

Acute retention. The patient reports that he has not been able to pass urine for several hours. The bladder is distended, causing considerable pain. In some cases the patient passes a small amount of urine continuously, without relief of the condition. Acute retention is more common in males than in females.

TREATMENT

Both trauma and medical conditions require transport to hospital. Treatment consists of:

- Taking a history
- Relief of pain
- Treatment of shock if present
- Transport to hospital
- Hand-over of information

Pain relief can be effected by use of Entonox (p. 132) and positioning. The patient should be allowed to find the most comfortable position.

Patients with acute retention may often say that they are going to pass urine. They should be reassured that this is normal and is no problem. It is unlikely that any urine will be passed but it is nevertheless a great source of anxiety.

Crush syndrome

When the circulation to a limb has been cut off for more than an hour, metabolites dangerous to the kidneys build up in the vascular system of the limb. If suddenly released this can lead to a rapid drop in blood pressure and damage to the kidneys. Try to ensure that pressure on a limb is relieved early in a rescue, even though it may not actually release the patient.

Medical supervision of fluid replacement therapy is essential in these cases.

Renal dialysis patients

Patients undergoing dialysis treatment will have a shunt positioned in the blood vessels of a limb. Figure 6.5 shows a typical shunt. There are two types of emergency that may result from the use of shunts, as described below.

Blood may clot in the shunt, requiring urgent transport to hospital. The shunt may accidentally be broken, allowing uncontrolled bleeding. In most cases the patient will be able to stop the bleeding without help. If the shunt has actually come out of the blood vessel, direct pressure and elevation of the limb will be necessary. Patients will carry a pneumatic cuff to use as a tourniquet if haemorrhage cannot be stopped by direct pressure.

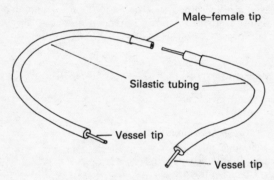

Fig. 6.5   An arteriovenous shunt.

Miscellaneous injuries

There is often little medical treatment to be carried out. The confidence of the patient, however, is all important. Often, second thoughts will make the patient unwilling to even admit to injury. Occasionally an ambulance has been called purely as an act of exhibitionism.

All patients in this category must be treated in a professional manner. Their confidence must be respected and no judgement or mockery should be detectable in the attitude of those treating the patient.

Transport

The pain associated with injury to the urogenital system limits the amount of vibration that patients will tolerate. Acute retention patients will often notice the smallest of bumps and will require a smooth ride.

7

Obstetrics

In the majority of cases childbirth proceeds naturally without intervention. The majority of mothers are healthy, as are their babies. Legally, all births must be attended by a midwife or doctor. On occasions only ambulance staff will be in attendance at the time, although a doctor or midwife should have been summoned to attend as soon as possible.

Ambulance staff must have sufficient knowledge of the relevant anatomy and procedures to attend a normal delivery, recognize problems and understand instructions from midwives and doctors.

ANATOMY

Anatomy of the female pelvis

The female bony pelvis differs from that of the male. The internal opening is rounded to allow as much room as possible for the passage of the fetus. Within the pelvis the uterus is attached by a number of ligaments (Fig. 7.1). The bladder, normally situated in the pelvis, can be forced up into the abdomen during pregnancy.

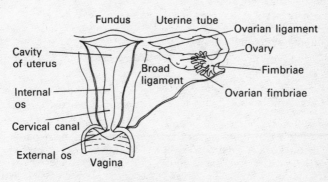

Fig. 7.1 Ligaments supporting the uterus.

119

Anatomy of the fetus

As the fetus develops in the uterus, the placenta, connected by the umbilical cord, carries out the functions of the lungs, intestines and kidneys. Following a normal birth anatomical changes take place to allow the infant to lead a separate existence.

The placenta.   The placenta, attached to the uterus, is part of the fetus. Circular in shape, it weighs approximately a sixth of the baby's birth weight. When seen after delivery the shiny fetal surface is visible. The maternal surface is rough with a thin layer of maternal decidua adhering.

The umbilical cord.   This may be from 1–200 centimetres long. The average length is 50 centimetres. It contains two arteries and one vein. At term the fetus is contained within three membranes: the maternal decidua lining the uterus, the chorion (of which the placenta is a specialist part) and the amnion, which forms the covering of the placenta and the cord. Within the amniotic sac is about 1200 millilitres of fluid—the liquor amnii.

Fetal circulation is shown in Figure 7.2. At birth, fetal carbon dioxide rises while the oxygen level falls. Respiration is stimulated and with the first breaths the ductus arteriosus closes. The foramen ovale closes in response to a rise in the left atrial pressure. Circulation in the cord stops when it is tied. This closes the ductus venosus. Likewise, the hypogastric arteries cease to function.

DELIVERY

Ambulance staff normally are involved with deliveries that are unexpectedly rapid, often to mothers with previous problem-free births. A normal delivery is cephalic—head first—facing the opposite direction to the mother.

Normal delivery

Signs and symptoms of labour are:

- A show—a small quantity of blood and mucus issuing from the vagina
- Contractions
- Cervical dilatation

In false labour, often associated with engagement of the head, the pains felt are at the front of the abdomen. True labour pains are felt at the back, travelling forward. The show is never present in false labour. Cervical dilatation can only be determined by vaginal examination which should not be attempted by ambulance personnel.

Normal delivery can be described in three stages (Fig. 7.3):

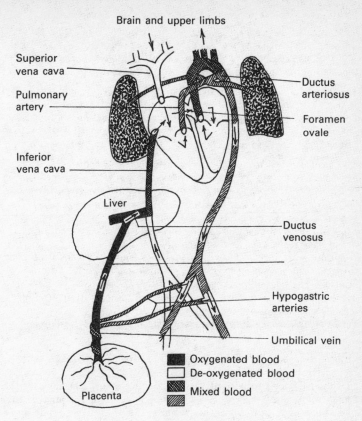

Fig. 7.2 The fetal circulation.

- Stage 1—the onset of true labour to full dilatation of the cervix. This normally coincides with rupture of the membranes.
- Stage 2—from full dilatation of the cervix until delivery of the child
- Stage 3—contraction of the uterus, expulsion of the placenta and further contraction to prevent bleeding

Stage 1. True labour is established with pains every 30 minutes (1/30). As contractions become more frequent they become more painful. If it is the mother's first baby (when the woman is known as a primipara) the first stage may last for up to 24 hours, but

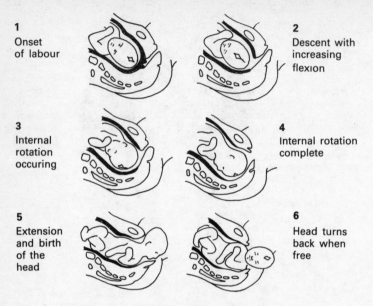

1
Onset
of labour

2
Descent with
increasing
flexion

3
Internal
rotation
occuring

4
Internal rotation
complete

5
Extension
and birth
of the
head

6
Head turns
back when
free

Fig. 7.3 The stages of a normal delivery.

more normally lasts for 8–10 hours. In multipara it will be considerably shorter.

It is safe for the patient to walk during stage 1 as long as the membranes have not ruptured. If they have, cord prolapse cannot be ruled out until a vaginal examination has been made by a qualified person. The patient should be kept semi-recumbent. A carry-chair should not be used. As the contractions become more painful, Entonox should be offered. Rubbing the patient's back can also give some relief.

Stage 2.   Contractions become stronger and more frequent. Starting at 1/5 they gradually increase in rate to 1/1 with only a few seconds between contractions. The mother wants to bear down and push with each contraction. To assist pushing, the mother should lie in a semi-recumbent position with her knees drawn up. (A recumbent position should be avoided because this could lead to pressure on the venae cavae from the unborn child, resulting in loss of consciousness.) She should take a deep breath, hold it and push. Pain relief with Entonox should be given throughout stage 2 if the mother so wishes.

Stage 2 lasts for about 1 hour but may be as short as 5 minutes.

As the widest diameter of the head is born—crowning—the birth must be controlled. This is done by telling the mother to pant with each contraction and not to push. A hand is placed on the baby's head and gentle pressure is applied. This pressure is released, but the hand is kept in place, at the end of a contraction, allowing a gradual, gentle birth. In this way tearing of the maternal perineum and brain haemorrhage in the child are avoided.

As the head is born a check is made to see if the cord is around the neck. If it is, and there is sufficient slack, it should be looped over the baby's head. **Do not pull on the cord**. If the cord is tight it should be clamped in two places and cut between the clamps (Fig. 7.4). Each of the baby's eyes should be cleaned with a separate, clean, moistened swab, wiping from the inside out.

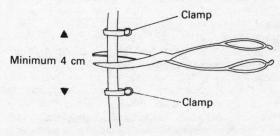

Fig. 7.4 Cutting the umbilical cord.

After the head is born the neck is flexed downwards to allow the birth of the upper shoulder. The head is then raised and the lower shoulder is born. The next contraction will deliver the body.

Take care—babies are slippery! Wrap the baby straightaway in a towel from the maternity pack and place it between the mother's legs. Clear the airway with a mucus extractor. It should cry at once and cyanosis should decrease. If not, start resuscitation immediately.

When the baby is breathing normally, place it on the mother's abdomen and transport them to hospital at normal speed.

Stage 3. After about 20 minutes contractions will restart. This signals stage 3 and the ambulance should be stopped. Do not pull on the cord; the placenta will deliver easily. The placenta should be saved for later examination. There will be a slight loss of blood, but any continuing loss should be treated as haemorrhage. The journey to hospital is resumed.

Practical considerations

When first seen the patient should be assessed. The following questions need to be answered:

- Is the patient in labour?
- At what stage is the labour and how frequent are the contractions?
- How many previous labours have there been and were there any problems?
- Have the membranes ruptured?
- How suitable is the present location of the patient for childbirth?

As a rule a patient should not be moved if the contractions are more frequent than 1/5. When contractions are 1/3 birth is imminent. It is better to deliver a baby in a house than in the cramped conditions of an ambulance.

Preparation

The patient needs to be reassured, kept warm and informed. One crew member at the head end talks to the mother and supervises pain relief. The other manages the delivery. Two blankets overlapping at the waist will allow ease of access whilst maintaining modesty. An incontinence pad under the patient aids clearing up afterwards and keeps the patient dry.

The attendant should wash his/her hands thoroughly. In an emergency Savlon rubbed into the skin is an alternative to alcohol hand rub. Surgical gloves are ideal but loose gloves add to the risk of dropping the child. Equipment should be laid out to hand but out of reach of splashes.

ABNORMAL CIRCUMSTANCES

Good antenatal care should provide advance warning of some abnormal circumstances. In many cases the patient will have notes available which will give some help, such as blood pressure readings and history of previous confinements.

Malpresentation/obstructed labour

Unless the baby is very small malpresentation will delay birth so that ambulance crews will rarely be involved with any other than normal deliveries. Figure 7.5 shows some of the more common malpresentations. As far as ambulance personnel are concerned there is specific treatment only for breech presentation. All other malpresentations will either deliver naturally or become obstructed. In the latter case urgent arrival at hospital is essential since the baby may well be distressed.

Breech delivery

This is commonly seen with twins where one is delivered cephalic and the other breech. In the emergency situation it is diagnosed by seeing the buttocks and anus or feet as the presenting part.

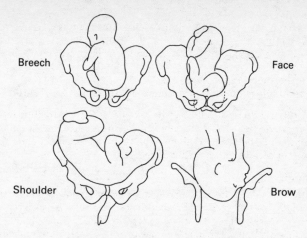

Breech

Face

Shoulder

Brow

Fig. 7.5 Common malpresentations.

The risks are tentorial tearing due to the sudden birth of the aftercoming head, fetal asphyxia due to nipping of the cord or premature breathing, and trauma caused by rough handling. Figure 7.6 shows a method of delivering a breech presentation. This should only be used in extreme circumstances when all attempts to get expert help have failed.

Haemorrhage

Haemorrhage is qualified by the stage at which it occurs:

- Before the twenty-eighth week, especially when the pregnancy is terminated, haemorrhage is termed 'abortion'.
- Bleeding after the twenty-eighth week and before the end of the second stage of labour termed 'antepartum haemorrhage' (APH).
- Haemorrhage after delivery is termed 'postpartum haemorrhage' (PPH).

Debate is taking place at the moment as to whether the 28-week period should be reduced to 26 weeks.

Abortion.   Figure 7.7 shows the different classifications of abortion. The majority proceed without catastrophic blood loss. Occasionally the patient will be severely shocked. Treatment is as for shock (see chapter 3), with good patient monitoring and assessment of blood loss. Some patients will complain of labour pains and Entonox can be used.

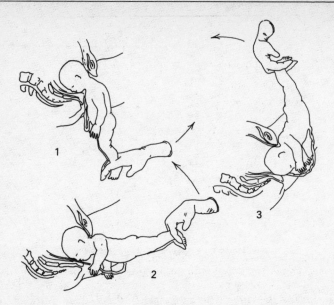

Fig. 7.6   The Burns–Marshall manoeuvre for breech delivery.

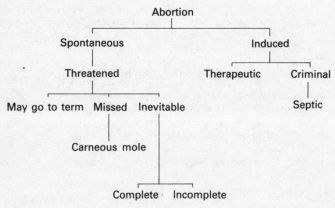

Fig. 7.7   The classification of abortion.

Antepartum haemorrhage.   This may be due to two causes:

- Placenta praevia (see Figure 7.8), where the placenta is below the fetus in the uterus. Thus it is squeezed by the fetus and if it comes away from the uterine wall, bleeding will occur.

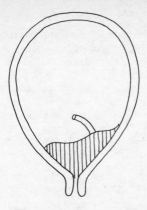

Fig. 7.8 Placenta praevia.

- Abruptio placenta, where bleeding is from a normally placed placenta. This may be due to high blood pressure or traumatic damage such as by a fall. Figure 7.9 shows the two types of abruptio placenta—concealed and revealed.

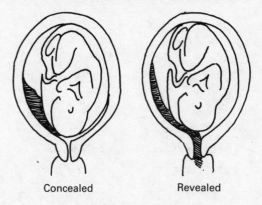

Concealed   Revealed

Fig. 7.9 Abruptio placentae.

Postpartum haemorrhage. This may occur up to 6 weeks after birth. It is most usually the result of infection or incomplete delivery of the placenta. Treatment can be carried out by a midwife or doctor, so it is essential to get aid to the patient or convey the patient, at the same time treating for shock.

Ectopic pregnancy

This is a misplaced pregnancy in the fallopian tubes. The lack of space leads to pain as the cells divide. If allowed to continue in the isthmus, the tube may rupture and severe bleeding into the peritoneum takes place.

Treatment for a ruptured ectopic pregnancy is that for shock (see chapter 3). The patient needs urgent hospital treatment. Those patients who have pain but no signs of shock should be transported in the semi-recumbent position. They may be more comfortable if the knees are drawn up. Shock following rupture may set in very rapidly. The patient should be monitored as frequently as possible.

Prolapsed cord

This is a serious condition which may lead to asphyxia of the fetus if pressure is allowed to bear on the cord. Diagnosis is either by a section of cord presenting at the vulva or being felt during vaginal examination by a qualified person.

Treatment is by placing the patient in the genupectoral position (Fig. 7.10). Gravity takes the weight of the fetus off the cord but does not prevent muscular action. For this reason the patient must be transported to hospital as soon as possible. A midwife or doctor can manually hold the pressure off the cord.

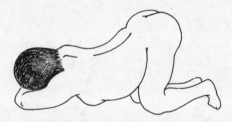

Fig. 7.10   The genupectoral position.

Eclampsia

From 28 weeks until 2 days after birth there is a risk of fits following a period of pre-eclampsia.

Signs and symptoms of pre-eclampsia are:

- Raised blood pressure
- Severe headaches
- Vomiting
- Oedema

- Epigastric pain
- Diminished urine output

Eclamptic fits may occur with no warning but usually follow pre-eclamptic signs and symptoms. There are four stages to a fit:

- Preliminary stage—where the eyes roll up, the face flushes and the muscles contract irregularly. This lasts for up to a minute.
- Tonic stage—half a minute during which the muscles are tensed. Cyanosis occurs as a result of the respiratory muscles being tensed.
- Clonic stage—violent muscle contractions, frothing at the mouth and snapping of the jaw, which lasts for 2–3 minutes.
- Coma stage—may be interrupted by further fits or by recovery. This stage may last for minutes or hours.

Treatment. This is as follows:

- Protect from injury during fit.
- Maintain airway. Remove false teeth and aspirate.
- Give oxygen.
- Reduce light level but be able to assess cyanosis.
- Reduce noise level. In a moving vehicle this can only be done by plugging the patient's ears with cotton wool or using ear defenders.
- Get the patient to specialist care without delay.

Emergency situations

Especially where patients have tried to conceal pregnancy from their family, birth may take place in difficult circumstances. Typically birth may have taken place into a lavatory pan. Each situation will be different but the following factors should be considered:

- The weight of the baby pulling on the cord should be avoided.
- The mother should be laid down as soon as possible.
- The baby should be resuscitated, kept warm and, when breathing, placed on the mother to benefit from her warmth.
- The cord should be clamped but not cut.
- If the mother is badly shocked her life takes precedence over that of the baby.

Premature birth

The definition of a premature baby is one that weighs 2500 grams or less. In addition, the length is under 45 centimetres and the skin is dull red, wrinkled and covered with downy hair. The bones of the skull are widely separated and the nails will not have grown to the ends of the nail beds. Most seriously, the baby may not be capable of effective breathing or temperature regulation.

Delivery will usually be easy but care should be taken to ensure that the birth is controlled. Resuscitation may be necessary and steps must be taken to keep the baby warm. Remember that the baby is not capable of producing heat so it must not be insulated from getting warm. The mother is the best heat source. Premature babies need specialist help as soon as possible.

8

Ambulance Aid Topics

PAIN RELIEF

Patients with a wide variety of conditions will suffer pain. Prolonged pain causes the body to produce catecholamines. These drugs produce vasoconstriction and reduced tissue perfusion contrary to the aims of resuscitation.

Pain relief not only benefits tissue perfusion but also prevents further damage caused by muscle contractions. The cooperation and assistance of a trapped patient can often be of help to rescuers.

There are four methods available to ambulance personnel by which pain can be relieved:

- Psychological—reassurance and an explanation of what is happening
- Practical—positioning, splinting and attention to needs
- Inhalation analgesia—Entonox
- Intravenous analgesia—obtaining medical aid to administer drugs

Psychological methods

The severity of pain is influenced by psychological factors. Pain tolerated throughout the day may become unbearable in the early hours of the morning when tiredness and loneliness help to increase perception.

In the case of trauma, patients are often concerned about other factors such as notifying relatives. Reassurance, allaying fears and getting action taken to solve patients' problems all help to minimize the pain they experience. Touch can be very comforting. Holding a patient's hand or touching their shoulder gives reassurance that help is at hand and often saves the need to talk.

Practical methods

Patients usually find the most comfortable position to suit themselves. However, some patients will need to be supported in position whilst others will require careful moving to achieve the best position.

Whilst the injuries will dictate how blankets are placed over a patient, most find the feeling of being wrapped up comforting.

Effective splinting gives good pain relief. Trapped patients may be held in what amounts to a splint. Extrication may therefore cause further pain as splinting is removed. Gentle sustained traction is effective in partially relieving the pain of limb fractures.

Patients can often give useful information about what is causing their discomfort. Not only is this useful in diagnosis but small adjustments of position can produce good pain relief.

Inhalation analgesia

Entonox, carried on UK ambulances since the early 1970s, is the trademark of Ohmeda Ltd. It is a 50% mixture of nitrous oxide and oxygen. Whilst mixed, inhalation produces raised tissue oxygenation at the same time as pain relief.

Pain relief from Entonox is as effective as narcotic analgesics. Its effect starts about 30 seconds after initial administration, giving greatest pain relief after about 2 minutes. The effect wears off about 2 minutes after stopping inhalation.

A demand regulator is used for administration. The patient uses a mask or mouthpiece and opens the valve with the negative pressure of inspiration. Where a mask is used it should have a clear area so that the patient's mouth can be seen at all times (Fig. 8.1).

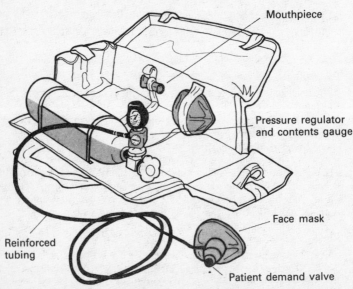

Mouthpiece

Pressure regulator and contents gauge

Face mask

Reinforced tubing

Patient demand valve

Fig. 8.1 The parts of an Entonox set.

The advantages of Entonox can be summarized as follows:

- Can be administered by ambulance personnel
- Gives rapid pain relief
- Does not mask symptoms
- Does not depress respiratory or heart function
- Is self administered by the patient
- Gives increased oxygen concentration
- No need to measure doses (self limiting as mask falls away)

At temperatures below −6°C nitrous oxide liquefies and separates from the oxygen, falling to the bottom of the cylinder. Although the oxygen given off first from such a cylinder will be safe, if ineffective, the nitrous oxide would be an asphyxiant.

Cylinders of Entonox exposed to temperatures below freezing and containing liquid should be immersed in warm water for 5 minutes and then inverted at least three times.

There are certain rules that must be followed for the administration of Entonox:

- **It must be self administered**. As the patient becomes drowsy the seal around the mask will break. In this way the patient controls the level of pain relief to suit his need.
- **The patient must be fully conscious**. Entonox is not required for unconscious casualties and should not be given if the patient cannot understand what is being offered.
- **Airway, Breathing and Circulation must be effective**. There is no benefit in relieving pain until basic stabilization has been achieved.

Entonox should not be administered to patients suffering from:

- Head injury
- Maxillofacial injury if the airway is not clear
- Pneumothorax
- The bends (compression sickness)
- The effects of drugs including alcohol
- Mental confusion

Safety precautions are as for oxygen (see chapter 3).

Intravenous analgesia

Ambulance personnel are not permitted to give intravenous drugs. However, on the rare occasions when Entonox is not suitable or effective on its own it should be recognized that pain relief is still needed. Medical aid, usually an immediate care doctor, should be summoned to administer the appropriate drugs.

POISONING

Poisoning occurs in a great variety of forms. In adults it is usually intentional, varying from an insignificant cry for help to lethal cocktails. Ambulance personnel are often confronted with a difficult domestic situation coupled with the need to compete against the clock. Management and detection skills are needed to obtain the necessary information. As with all ambulance work the hand-over is important. Treatment in hospital will, in many cases, be based on the information obtained by the crew.

Poisons

Any substance which has a harmful effect on the body is a poison. The substance may be in the form of a gas, liquid or solid. Entry into the body may be by:

- Ingestion—swallowing tablets, eating plants or berries
- Inhalation—breathing car exhaust fumes, sewer gas or toxic gases from a house fire
- Injection—controlled drugs, snake bites
- Skin absorption—handling certain explosives or creosote

Diagnosis

In the emergency situation the diagnosis of poisoning has usually been made before the call. The majority of patients show few symptoms initially. The call may be made by someone who discovers evidence or by a patient who regrets having taken an overdose.

The information required is:

- What has been taken?
- How much has been taken?
- With what was it taken?
- When was it taken?
- What proof is there?
- Has the patient vomited?

Proof is necessary because there is often confusion and sometimes the patient may lie. Proof usually takes the form of containers or discarded tablets found at the scene.

Tracking down what has been taken must also include what might have been taken. For example, a patient with two half-empty bottles of tablets may have taken some of each, despite what he says.

Although there should be no unnecessary delay, time spent getting the facts correct at the scene is well spent.

Before treatment can commence it is important to identify poisoning by corrosive substances or petroleum derivatives.

Table 4. Patterns of poisoning.

Pattern	Poisons commonly involved
Coma, hypotension, flaccidity	Benzodiazepines Barbiturates Alcohol Opioids Beta-blocking drugs Many others
Coma, hyperreflexia, tachycardia, dilated pupils	Tricyclic antidepressants Anticholinergic agents Phenothiazines
Malaise, restlessness, nausea, weakness	Carbon monoxide Addictive states and withdrawal Solvents Insecticides Lead, mercury, arsenic
Behavioural disturbances	Psychotropic drugs Adverse effects of drugs, e.g. steroids Addictive states and withdrawal Solvent abuse LSD *Psilocybe* mushroom
Burns in mouth, dysphagia, abdominal pain, distension	Corrosives Caustics Paraquat

Corrosives leave burns in or around the mouth; petroleum derivatives can be smelt on the breath.

A number of garden, indoor and hedgerow plants are poisonous. However, most are bitter and cases of poisoning are rare. Ensure that a large enough sample of the plant is taken for positive identification.

Tropical snakes may be encountered at ports, but the adder is the only poisonous snake endemic to the British Isles. Positive identification is required before treatment can commence at hospital.

Patterns of poisoning

There are certain patterns of signs and symptoms that help to diagnose poisoning agents (Table 4). It is important to look for and report these to the hospital. Signs and symptoms to be monitored are:

- Level of consciousness
- Muscle tone
- Skin changes
- Pupils
- Temperature
- Breath odour
- Blood pressure
- Convulsions
- Respiratory function
- Cardiac arrhythmias

Treatment

Many patients will show no symptoms of poisoning. Whilst there is any doubt that poisoning has taken place, these patients must be assumed to be at risk. The following steps should be taken for treatment:

- Remove the patient from contact with the poison (if possible).
- Check and clear the airway.
- Assess the vital signs: pulse, respiration and pupils.
- Resuscitate the patient if required.
- Place the patient in the recovery position.
- Collect the evidence of poisoning.
- Transport the patient.

Always approach with care. Where a patient has been poisoned by an inhaled poison, the risk may be as great for the rescuer. Having removed the patient to fresh air, use 100% oxygen. Remember that exhaled air resuscitation must not be used in cases of poisoning by agents that may in turn poison the rescuer. These include caustic substances and highly poisonous gases such as cyanide.

Poisoning by a skin-absorbed agent requires immediate washing with water. If a large area is involved it may be necessary to use a hose. Warm water is more effective at removing chemicals such as phenols. However, there must be no delay in treatment.

Obtain the history as early as possible. The patient may become unconscious at any time.

Induction of vomiting is not recommended for the following reasons:

- Methods of inducing vomiting can:
  1 cause added complications—salt water
  2 delay transport to hospital—syrup of ipecacuanha
  3 be dangerous to ambulance personnel—pharyngeal stimulation with the fingers

- Vomiting may cause considerable danger to the patient's airway due to suppression of the cough reflex.
- Corrosive substances will cause further damage to the mouth and pharynx.
- Petroleum derivatives, especially in children, may cause damage to the respiratory tract if aspirated.

Where distance from hospital results in long journey times the use of activated charcoal as an absorbant may be of use. At present this is not generally accepted by ambulance services but should be investigated.

A conscious patient who has ingested a corrosive poison should be given water or milk to drink. If available, without delay, ice cream is beneficial since the cold temperature slows absorption and peristalsis.

Oxygen should be given for hypoxia. This may be due to gas or smoke poisoning or may be secondary to other poisons. In all cases a clear airway and a good minute volume must be ensured before oxygen therapy is commenced. Paraquat poisoning is an absolute contraindication to the administration of oxygen.

Snake bite. In cases of snake bite or accidental injection, treatment aims to prevent the circulation of poison in the blood stream. The patient should be carried and not allowed to walk. The affected limb may be splinted if this helps to prevent movement. No pressure should be applied to the wound.

Transport

Patients who have been poisoned tolerate transport well. Time is important and there should be no avoidable delay in reaching hospital. The ride must be safe and the attendant must be able to accurately assess his patient.

Travel sickness is common, especially where tablets and alcohol have been taken. As long as the airway is protected and the poison is not corrosive, this does little harm. Stomach contents should be retained for analysis at hospital.

MENTAL ILLNESS

Mental illness is a loose definition. It is applied to illnesses that affect the mind rather than the body. Often, severe illness of the body may affect the mind and vice versa. There are a number of terms that need to be defined:

- Psychosis—a mental disorder that affects the whole personality. The patient is unaware that he is acting this way and has lost touch with reality.

- Neurosis—the patient is aware that something is wrong and indeed may be very worried by it.
- Mental subnormality—usually a congenital condition, where the development of intelligence has been arrested. There may or may not also be physical handicap.
- Psychopathy—a persistent disorder of the mind which results in abnormally aggressive or seriously irresponsible conduct on the part of the patient.
- Depression—a melancholy frame of mind. This ranges from a mood that everyone occasionally experiences to total apathy or suicidal tendencies.
- Mania—an excessively high mood. The patient may in extreme cases become physically exhausted.
- Delusions—false beliefs that cannot be corrected by reasoning. These beliefs may be pleasant to the patient but most cause distress.
- Hallucinations—apparent physical experience of something which is not there. Hearing and seeing are the senses most commonly involved.
- Phobia—an irrational fear of things or situations. It may be so severe as to be a handicap to normal life.
- Compulsive behaviour—a need to repeat pointless patterns of behaviour in a certain way.
- Paranoid delusions—delusions in which the patient feels persecuted.

Working with the mentally ill

Patients cannot be talked out of their mental state. To do so leads to argument and will upset the patient.

Do not enter into the patient's delusions or hallucinations. To confirm their experiences only adds to the problem.

Be sincere and try not to enter into a discussion about the patient's problems.

If the patient wants to talk, listen. If the patient does not talk, don't force conversation.

Do not lie to the patient. This will only destroy what little faith the patient has in reality.

The use of force

The Mental Health Act (chapter 9) allows for the use of force, in certain cases, to get a patient to go to hospital. Force must only be used as a last resort. A firm, kindly approach with no sign of rush often results in acceptance by the patient.

Violent patients

Patients become violent for a variety of reasons. Some are suffering from mental illness, others from reaction to drugs. Increasingly, ambulance personnel are involved with violent incidents which require careful impartial handling.

Experience is the most important factor in successfully dealing with a violent incident, but the following points should be noted:

- Never assume that people are going to be violent until they are. Such an assumption may provoke a reaction.
- Do not lose your temper. Maintain a professional attitude—firm and friendly.
- Don't dare the patient and never whisper in sight of the patient.
- Always have plenty of time; don't appear to rush. Be aware of the danger to people but don't worry about property.

If, despite all efforts, violence results, there are several steps that should be taken to protect the patient and others from harm:

Good preparation

- Ensure that there are sufficient people to cope.
- Employ medical assistance if appropriate.
- Know the terrain and remove potential dangers.
- Check yourself for dangers, e.g. scissors.
- Position and clear the vehicle.
- Clear other people from the scene.
- Agree on a plan of action beforehand.

Physical restraint

- Only use as a last resort.
- Attempt to reduce aggression.
- Don't rush at the patient.
- Hold him only near the major joints.
- Never hold the head or neck.
- Avoid pressure on the chest or abdomen.
- Be close to or far away from the patient to avoid being hit.

The best restraint is a blanket wrapped around the patient. It provides good control without appearing aggressive either to the patient or to bystanders.

Where elderly patients become violent, special care must be taken. The bones and skin of elderly patients are more fragile and there is a great risk of damage.

Suicidal patients must never be left alone. Be prepared for a considerable degree of cunning amongst these patients. The chief danger is allowing access to a room where the patient can lock himself in.

Self protection. Handling violent people is dangerous. Help is always available and in many cases it is best to hang back until it arrives. Above all, the golden rule is 'Don't become a casualty yourself'.

DIABETES MELLITUS

Diabetes is a disorder of carbohydrate metabolism associated with a lack of insulin. Insulin is required for cells to use glucose. Thus, if insulin levels are low, the blood sugar level rises—hyperglycaemia. Lack of sugar—hypoglycaemia—results from an overdosage of insulin or insufficient carbohydrate intake.

Signs and symptoms

Hypoglycaemia	*Hyperglycaemia*
• Rapid onset of signs and symptoms	• Gradual onset of symptoms
• Headache	• Abdominal pain and vomiting
• Aggressive, may appear drunk	• Restless and confused
• Unconsciousness	• Unconsciousness
• -Full, rapid pulse	• Air hunger
• Skin pale, cold, clammy	• Weak, rapid pulse
• Copious saliva	• Breath smells of acetone

It is notoriously difficult to distinguish the reasons for unconsciousness in these cases. Signs and symptoms often do not give a clear picture. A history of the pattern of meals and medication, needle marks, identification bracelets and sugar lumps in the pocket usually provides the information that the patient is a diabetic. Where there is doubt over the level of blood sugar, the reaction of the patient to the administration of oral sugar solution gives a good indication. With low blood sugar beneficial results will be seen in minutes.

Treatment

If the patient is conscious he will often know what is required. Diabetics usually carry sugar for such events. A glass of water or milk with a heaped tablespoon of sugar will often stabilize the condition. The patient should see a doctor soon afterwards to determine whether further treatment is required.

Nothing should be given by mouth to an unconscious patient. However, a small amount of glucose rubbed into the gums may be enough for the patient to regain consciousness. There are now proprietary gels available for this purpose.

For the deeply unconscious patient, rapid transport to hospital is necessary. Serious brain damage may be caused by delay.

DISORDERS OF HEAT AND COLD

Normal body temperature is about 37°C, rising and falling slightly in relation to the time of day. This temperature is maintained by the body so that the chemical reactions of the metabolism can proceed at a constant rate. Heating and cooling of the body activates compensatory systems. However, if these systems fail to maintain the core temperature, there will be a serious effect on the working of the body (Fig. 8.2).

Temperature regulation

The heat-regulating centre situated in the cerebrum, coupled with the vasomotor centre in the medulla oblongata, effect control over the body temperature.

Heat is produced by several processes:

- Voluntary muscles—contraction produces heat
- Shivering—an involuntary muscle action
- The liver—a by-product of metabolism
- The digestive organs—muscular contraction and metabolism

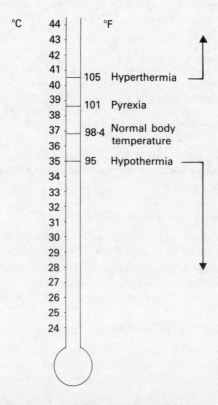

Fig. 8.2 Temperature conversion.

Heat is lost from the body by:

- Evaporation—sweat or water in clothing draws heat from the skin as it evaporates.
- Radiation—any uninsulated part of the body radiates heat.
- Conduction—heat passes into clothing and other contacts with the body.
- Convection—heat rises, setting up air currents that take heat from the body.

Certain factors control the rate of heat loss. The difference between the body temperature and the environment is termed the 'temperature gradient'. The greater the temperature gradient, the more rapid the heat loss.

Wind combined with cold can accelerate cooling. The presence of wet clothing, allowing water to evaporate in the wind, aggravates the problem still further. The wind chill factor goes up by the square of the wind speed. Thus, doubling the wind speed increases cooling by four times.

Exposure to heat

It takes several weeks for the body to adjust to a hot climate. For this reason people in temperate climates are susceptible to problems of heat when the weather suddenly changes. Activity aggravates the problem, so generally patients are fit, healthy and young. Hot working conditions, especially in confined spaces, may cause problems. There are a number of complaints from which these people may suffer:

Heat syncope. Vasodilatation, in an effort to cool the body, causes low blood pressure. This causes the patient to faint.

Heat exhaustion. Water loss over a period of time leads to dehydration. In extreme cases this can lead to a condition resembling hypovolaemic shock.

Salt depletion. This results in exhaustion, nausea and vomiting brought about by a loss of salt in sweat.

Heat stroke. Excessive heating causes the failure of the thermo-regulatory system, and the core temperature rises. The patient becomes unconscious and does not sweat, despite having a high body temperature.

Treatment. This is as follows:

- Remove the patient to a cool place.
- If the patient is unconscious, maintain the airway.
- Wrap the patient in a wet sheet and fan him vigorously.
- If the patient is conscious, encourage him to sip water.
- If cramps are present, salt added to fruit juice is beneficial.

Exposure to cold

Hypothermia affects a wide variety of people. The condition is caused in several different ways:

- Inadequate energy production (seen in babies and in the elderly)
- Excessive heat loss
  1 Rapid—immersion in cold water
  2 Slow—hill-walkers out for the day
  3 Very slow—the elderly with insufficient heating

Signs and symptoms are shown in Figure 8.3. It should be noted that the only reliable way to diagnose hypothermia is to use a low reading thermometer to ascertain the body temperature.

Hypothermia is often found with other injuries, the cause of hypothermia being the inability of the patient to move and keep warm.

Treatment. Peripheral circulation shuts down when the body is cold, keeping warm blood circulating around the vital organs of the body core. Rewarming at the wrong rate may have disastrous effects as vasodilatation rapidly takes place.

Rewarming should be at the same speed at which cooling took place. Thus, immersion hypothermia, if the casualty is still

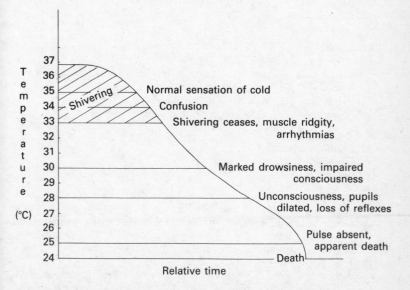

Fig. 8.3 The progression of hypothermia—signs and symptoms.

conscious, can be treated by getting the patient to take vigorous exercise.

For the more normal slow-onset hypothermia treatment aims to:

- Prevent further heat loss
- Prevent evaporation by removing wet clothing
- Allow the patient to absorb heat gradually from the environment

Note must be taken of the temperature gradient. When first found in a cold environment the patient will benefit from insulation such as a space blanket covered by a conventional blanket. This will retain what little heat there is as well as the small amount of heat being produced. Later, when the patient has been moved to a warm ambulance, the temperature gradient has been reversed. Now insulation must be removed to allow the heat to reach the patient.

Heat is lost underneath the patient as well as on top. A patient lying on the floor will benefit from a blanket underneath him as well as on top. Especially elderly patients cannot tolerate the weight of too many blankets; in extreme circumstances their breathing may be affected. Covering the extremities and the head, not the face, usually proves to be most comfortable for the patient.

Death is difficult to determine in a patient suffering from hypothermia, especially in the elderly. Therefore, attempts at resuscitation should be continued as long as possible or until medical opinion can be sought.

BURN AND SCALD INJURIES

Burn and scald injuries occur both in the home and the workplace. Such injuries are very emotive and require considerable skill to deal with the patient as well as bystanders.

The injury may be caused by one of the following:

- Thermal agents
- Chemical agents
- Radiated heat
- Electricity

A burn or scald is an injury affecting the skin and deeper tissues. The skin varies in thickness in different parts of the body. For example, on the dorsum of the hand or foot it is thin, whereas on the sole of the foot or the palm of the hand it is thick. Therefore, a burn to the dorsum of the hand may be a lot deeper relatively than a burn to the palm of the hand.

Burns may be 'full thickness', with complete destruction of the skin and sometimes of the underlying tissues. Alternatively, damage may be of 'partial thickness', with blistering or merely erythema (reddening of the skin).

Thermal agents

This term covers the wide extremes of temperature that can cause a range of injuries from extreme heat to extreme cold. The commonest thermal injury is the scald suffered by a child upsetting a kettle or teapot over itself. About 12% of scald injuries to children are from this cause.

One fluid ounce or 28 millilitres of liquid covers 500 square centimetres of skin. Remember also that a 1% scald to an adult equates to about a 9% scald in a child.

Flame burns. A box of matches may be left lying around by an unsuspecting parent and may be found and used by children. Clothing, furniture or paper may be ignited. Gas appliances may explode causing burns from the flame and respiratory damage from the ensuing blast. Chip-pan fires may cause injury either from the flames or from the hot fat. Flames in house fires, with modern furnishings, may be less of a danger than the toxic gases given off (see p. 48).

Flammable liquids. Injuries involving flammable liquids are mostly found in industrial or occupational accidents. The area of the body involved tends to be extensive because of the explosive nature of flammable substances which enable clothing to catch fire easily. Burns may also occur from butane or propane cylinders used on the camp-site or in the blow-lamp.

Contact burns. An alert adult does not usually catch hold of hot objects deliberately. However, the elderly patient who suffers a stroke or an epileptic fit may stay in contact with a hot object long enough to sustain a burn. Hot-water bottles should never be used with elderly or immobile patients. Children crawling around the house whilst exploring become fascinated with red-hot electric fire elements. Catching hold of them, they may sustain not only a burn but also an electric shock.

Especially in the industrial situation burns may result from substances such as tar or molten plastic which set in place on the skin.

Chemical agents

The concentration of the chemical, the duration of contact and its chemical reaction with the tissues will determine the extent of damage. Acids will coagulate the surface tissues, become neutralized and create their own barrier to deeper penetration. Alkalis penetrate deeper and have a more prolonged effect. Some chemicals, such as lime, only burn when mixed with water.

Radiated heat

It is normal to sunbathe wearing the minimum of clothing, so sunburn may be extensive. Although blistering may not be visible initially, loss of body fluid may occur, leading to shock and dehydration. Sunburn is painful and should never be treated as a trivial injury.

Another source of radiated heat is domestic fires. People who stand with their back to the fire can become burnt without damage to their clothing.

Electrical burns

The severity of injury depends on many factors such as:

- Amperage
- Voltage
- Tissue resistance
- Area of contact
- Duration of contact

High voltage burns.   Contact with high-voltage electric power lines in the order of 30 000 volts causes extensive burning and may involve traumatic amputation of parts of limbs.

Low voltage burns.   Injury may appear less severe but there may be hidden damage to structures along the track taken by the current. The patient may have fallen from a height or suffered violent muscular contractions, possibly causing the dislocation or fracture of limbs. A sudden flash may result in blindness or arc eye injuries.

Treatment

The priorities of treatment are:

- Personal safety of rescuers
- History of the accident
- Cooling of burns
- Resuscitation
- Assessment
- To prevent possible entry of infection
- To prevent further loss of body heat
- Constant reassurance
- Relief of pain

Assessment

The Wallace rule of nines can be used to assess the amount of body area burnt. Figure 8.4 shows how the rule of nines is applied.

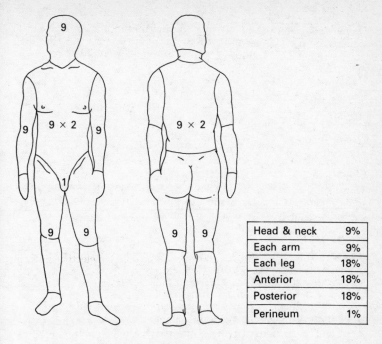

Head & neck	9%
Each arm	9%
Each leg	18%
Anterior	18%
Posterior	18%
Perineum	1%

Fig. 8.4   Wallace's rule of nines.

All burnt areas are included, whether partial or full thickness. Only erythema is ignored. Alternatively, a quick assessment can be made by using the size of the patient's hand with closed fingers to represent 1% of his body area.

If the burn is more than 15% in the adult or more than 5–10% in the child, it is important that intravenous fluids are commenced early. The classical signs of shock are not always present in the first hour. In hospital, careful measurement of fluids will be undertaken and large quantities should not be given early on. Setting up an intravenous infusion whilst it is still possible can save a great deal of trouble. However, accessible veins in good condition may be at a premium and therefore, if in doubt, do not proceed.

Body heat

Loss of skin causes difficulty to the patient in controlling his body temperature. For instance, no sweating will take place from burnt areas.

Clothing

Flames must be extinguished by smothering with a blanket. Cold water must then be used to cool the burnt area until loose clothing can be removed. Clothing adhering to the skin should be left in place.

Clothing over scald injuries should be removed since it holds hot liquid for some time against the skin.

If possible, remove rings and bracelets from hands and arms before swelling starts.

Cooling may have to go on for some time to cool a deep burn. Cooling can often be continued during transport to hospital.

Chemicals

These should be washed off with copious amounts of water. For some chemicals there are specific solutions to use. Do not delay by waiting for their arrival: use water at first.

Electricity

Isolate the supply—do not become another victim. In extreme circumstances it may be necessary to move the patient from the supply with, for example, a wooden pole. Even this should not be attempted with high voltage supplies.

Hot smoke or steam

A patient who has been in a confined space with hot smoke or steam may have sustained burns to his respiratory tract (see chapter 3).

The relief of pain

Pain is due to the stimulation of numerous nerve endings in the damaged skin. It is more severe in superficial burns. In the deeper burn there is extensive destruction of the nerve endings so that these burns may be relatively painless. Pain can be relieved in several ways:

- Immersion in cold water. Take care when placing an infant in a cold bath that he does not become hypothermic
- Covering with clean towels soaked in water
- Entonox, provided that there are no airway burns and that the level of consciousness is not impaired

Dressings

There are several different dressings available to cover burns:

- Roehampton type foam dressings—can become soaked in exudate, providing entry for infection and allowing heat loss

- Polythene bags—can be used for hands
- Cling film—if put on tight can constrict swelling tissues
- Dry sterile burn sheets—when applied become wet and provide an avenue for infection and heat loss

At present there is no perfect dressing for ambulance use in cases of burns. Sterile space blankets may provide the answer after further research.

Reassurance

The patient will need help. He will be feeling dazed, shocked, upset and distressed. He may feel that he will be permanently disfigured. If a child is involved then parents or other relatives often feel guilty, blaming themselves, or downright aggressive as though it is everyone else's fault. Ambulance personnel must take charge of the situation, be confident and provide reassurance.

Mortality due to burns

The mortality rate depends on two main factors:

- The percentage of the body surface burned
- The age of the patient

A general rule of thumb is, if the percentage body surface area burned added to the age of the patient is more than 100, then death is likely.

For example:

Percentage burn	= 30%	
Age of patient	= 76	
Total	= 106 (death is likely)	
Percentage burn	= 30%	
Age of patient	= 20	
Total	= 50 (recovery is likely)	

Deaths are usually due to complications of the burning injury. Primarily, these are infection and fluid loss.

Other injuries

A victim of a burning incident may have other injuries. Treatment of burns must not be allowed to interfere with the diagnosis and treatment of other possibly more urgent injuries.

9

Health, Hygiene and Infection Control

WHAT CAUSES AN INFECTION?

Every day we come into contact with literally millions of minute living microorganisms. Fortunately, most of these do no harm at all, but a few, given the right circumstances, can and do cause disease. Microorganisms capable of causing disease are referred to as pathogens. The commonest pathogens to cause disease in man are bacteria and viruses.

WHAT IS AN INFECTION?

Infection is the state of ill-health which occurs when a sufficient number of virulent pathogenic microorganisms invade a vulnerable site in the host and cause either a localized sepsis, for example a septic finger, or a generalized illness, for example influenza.

WHERE DOES INFECTION COME FROM?

Although some infections in this country can be transmitted from birds and animals, most infections in man come from man. Communicability usually depends upon a chain of events, but most important to consider is the site of the infection in the host. For example, an infection of the gastrointestinal tract causing diarrhoea is unlikely to be breathed into the air when the patient talks or coughs. However, the infecting microorganism will be excreted in the faeces and will readily contaminate the hands, bed linen and any other equipment or material that has been in contact with the patient.

HOW IS INFECTION SPREAD?

Microorganisms cannot walk or fly and have to be carried from one position to another. Infection can be spread by direct or indirect contact with the source. Most commonly, transfer is by direct contact via the hands of the carer who is handling or nursing the patient. However, infection can also spread by indirect contact via contaminated equipment, material, food and water supplies; or by the air-borne route in dust or in droplets caused by coughs or sneezes.

PROTECTION AGAINST DISEASE

The healthy person's body is generally able to defend itself against many diseases by its own defence mechanisms. The body has several types of defence mechanism. The skin and mucous membranes act as a physical barrier and, together with the chemical enzymes such as those found in tears and secretions, act as a first line of defence to invading microorganisms. The bloodstream, which acts as a second line of defence, contains highly active white cells which either destroy or neutralize the invading pathogens. These neutralizing cells are known as the 'immune system'.

Immunity is the degree of resistance to a disease which may be naturally or artificially acquired. Naturally acquired immunity may be inherited from the mother at birth, giving the baby protection for a short time from specific diseases, or it may be induced when the person has had the disease and the body has produced its own defences in the bloodstream known as antibodies, for example childhood illnesses such as measles and chickenpox. Antibodies may also be artificially acquired by immunization and vaccination against certain diseases. Many ambulance personnel will be immune against the common infectious diseases, having had them in childhood, and will have been immunized or vaccinated against certain specific diseases. It is important, however, to make sure that their immunizations are up to date as they do not necessarily confer life-long immunity. The occupational health department will normally be responsible for advising staff of their status.

INFECTIOUS DISEASES

Table 5 shows infectious diseases divided into three classes:

- **Class 1** diseases are not considered to be a cross-infection risk for ambulance personnel handling such cases, e.g. malaria cases, or precautions are not considered necessary as they would not afford adequate protection, e.g. influenza cases.
- **Class 2** diseases require the following standard precautions:

  1 Personnel should have available disposable impermeable protective clothing.

2 Disposable gloves and aprons should be worn when there is a possibility of contact with body secretions from infectious patients.

Services will have their own procedures which may vary slightly from those above.

- **Class 3** contains those exotic diseases which require handling by a specialist team. Procedures are laid down in each service for this purpose.

PREVENTING AND CONTROLLING INFECTION

Many infections can be prevented or controlled by understanding what causes infection, learning ways in which microorganisms transfer, and adhering to infection control policies and procedures applicable in your service.

Personal care and hygiene

Personal care and hygiene are important because they help to ensure a fit and healthy body. Poor personal care can lead to a vulnerability to infection and illness, social isolation, loss of self-respect and respect of patients. Personal care and hygiene mean a regular routine involving daily washing, eating a balanced diet and getting enough rest and exercise.

Daily washing

The skin is the first line of defence to invading microorganisms. It also helps to regulate the body temperature and eliminates waste by sweating. Skin needs to be washed and cared for regularly. How often you need a bath or shower depends on your type of skin and the job you have been involved in. Most people should bath or shower daily. After bathing or showering, always rinse the skin well from soap residues and then dry thoroughly to remove all moisture, especially between the toes and the buttocks. Use a moisturizer for dry skin, especially on the hands in winter to avoid cracking.

Hair

Hair and scalp can usually be kept healthy with careful and frequent care. Hair should be brushed daily to stimulate the hair and scalp and spread the natural oils, and washed regularly, the frequency of washing depending on the type of hair. A shampoo once a week will normally suffice for dry hair, whilst greasy hair may need washing up to two or three times a week. Remember to wash the brush and comb when washing the hair.

Teeth

Care of the mouth helps to prevent tooth decay, gum problems

Table 5. Infectious diseases and precautions required.

Class 1—no specific protective precautions
          Bronchiolitis of infants
          Bronchitis
          Conjunctivitis in an adult/infant of whatever cause
†   Diphtheria
          Gas gangrene
          Glandular fever
          Impetigo
          Influenza
          Legionellosis
          Malaria
*   Measles
**   Meningitis/encephalitis
*   Mumps
          Pneumonia
          Puerperal sepsis
*†   Rubella
          Tetanus
†   Tuberculosis
          Tonsillitis
†   Whooping cough
†   Polio

Class 2—standard precautions
*   Chickenpox
          Cholera
          Diarrhoea/enteritis of whatever cause
          Erysipelas
†   Hepatitis (jaundice) of whatever cause
*   Herpes zoster (shingles) syndrome
          Human immune deficiency syndrome (AIDS)
          Leptospirosis

Class 3—to be handled by a specialist team
          Lassa fever
          Marburg/Ebola virus
          Plague
          Rabies
          Smallpox

* Where possible, ambulance personnel who are known to be immune, that is have had the disease, should handle the patient. Ambulance personnel known to be immune need not wear protective clothing when handling patients with chickenpox. Neither need protective clothing be worn when handling patients with herpes zoster if ambulance personnel are known to be immune from chickenpox.

** Various types of meningitis are infectious, but none are very readily transferred by casual contact such as transporting the patient from home to hospital by ambulance. If, however, exhaled air resuscitation has been given, the medical team in care of the patient should be informed. Prophylactic antibiotics may be given.

† Ambulance personnel should be immunized/vaccinated against these infections.

and bad breath. Bacteria in the mouth form plaque. This is a substance which sticks to teeth, and if allowed to build up on the teeth, damages the gums and loosens the teeth. Teeth should be brushed at least twice a day with toothpaste or powder. Visit the dentist regularly every 6 months for an examination.

Balanced diet

Good nutrition is essential to overall health. A balanced diet should contain a daily intake of a variety of food, which includes the following types:

- **Protein** for building and repairing body cells and tissues
- **Carbohydrates** for energy
- **Fats** for reserve energy (choose polyunsaturated fats and oils)
- **Mineral salts** for healthy cell activity
- **Water** to maintain water balance
- **Roughage** to stimulate bowel excretion

Rest and exercise

Keeping physically fit is also a part of personal care and hygiene. The amount of exercise depends on the individual. Driving law specifies the hours it is permissible to work, and it is important that the time off is actually used to rest. Shift work can be disturbing to sleep patterns but sufficient exercise will aid relaxation.

INFECTION CONTROL AND THE ENVIRONMENT

To make the environment of an ambulance safe by sterilization would be almost impossible, nor is it necessary. The rational approach is to consider the infection risks, evaluate the nature and degree of known or suspected contamination, and consider the possible and probable contact with the patient.

Direct spread of microorganisms from the floor, the sides of the ambulance and its fittings is unlikely although cleanliness of the ambulance is an important factor in the control of infection. A thorough cleaning with a freshly prepared detergent solution, changed as necessary, is, in the vast majority of circumstances, the only necessary requirement of decontamination of the ambulance. Disposable cloths should be used for cleaning surfaces, and mops with a washable or disposable head should be used for the floor. An efficient household cleanser removes the nutrients required for the growth and survival of microorganisms, and cleaning physically removes many of them. Surfaces should be left as dry as possible as many microorganisms die when dry. Surfaces accidently contaminated with organic matter such as blood, pus or faeces provide an ideal growth medium for microorganisms and should be cleaned up as soon as possible. Contamination should be removed with paper towels, whilst wearing unsterile disposable gloves, discarded into a waste sack and finally the surface washed down with an environmental disinfectant containing a detergent or detergent properties (see below).

The application of a fine spray of a chemical disinfectant—'fogging'—to the inside of an ambulance for disinfection is usually unsatisfactory and not recommended. There is no evidence that this means of disinfection has any advantage over a thorough domestic clean using a chemical disinfectant and detergent.

Formaldehyde for terminal disinfection of the inside of an ambulance may, under rare circumstances for specific infections under the category of exotic diseases, be recommended. If formaldehyde is used it is only effective under optimum conditions of high temperature and humidity and the windows and doors of the ambulance have to be adequately sealed.

Disinfection by other gases such as sulphur dioxide are thoroughly unreliable and not recommended.

After carrying patients with a known or suspected infectious disease, ambulances should be washed and cleaned as described below before transporting another patient.

Disinfection

Cleaning is a form of disinfection. Cleaning physically removes many microorganisms, but in certain cases of gross contamination or known infection it is advisable to have the added protection of a chemical disinfectant. Disinfection is not expected to kill all microorganisms but will, if accurately diluted, destroy the majority of vegetative organisms. Chemical disinfectants should be freshly diluted immediately before use and discarded after use.

Disinfectants commonly used.   These are as follows:

Clear soluble phenolics (CSP)
This is a relatively cheap, useful environmental disinfectant which is active against a wide range of bacteria, fungi and some viruses. It is not readily neutralized by organic matter. However it does, if used over a long period, tend to affect rubber and certain plastic surfaces by making them brittle and/or increasing porosity. CSPs are usually recommended to be used at a 1% dilution.

Hypochlorites (bleach)
Hypochlorites, particularly sodium hypochlorite (NaDcc) in tablet form, are convenient to store and easy to dilute accurately. NaDcc is not readily inactivated by organic matter and has the added advantage that an anionic detergent can be added to the solution. Hypochlorite at a 10 000 p.p.m. 1% dilution is effective against

hepatitis B virus and human immunodeficiency virus (responsible for AIDS). At 1000 p.p.m. 0.1% it can be used as a general purpose disinfectant for known or suspected contaminated areas.

Sterilization

Sterilization is a process which destroys all known forms of living microorganisms. Sterilization is necessary for equipment or material which comes into contact or which is introduced into normally sterile sites.

Much commercially available equipment has been sterilized by ionizing radiation and stamped with an expiry date and shelf-life. This date should always be checked before use since out-of-date stock, although remaining sterile if the packaging is undamaged, may have degraded and become unsafe. Many soft packs of dressings and packs sterilized by autoclaving (sterilizing by steam under pressure) at local hospitals may no longer be dated. This is because packs do not become gradually less sterile so, provided the pack remains undamaged, it is safe to use.

Sterile packs should be stored, ready for use, in a clean, dry environment. Paper and plastic bags can be used as dust covers.

The cleaning, disinfection and sterilization of patient equipment

Microbial contamination of patient equipment, like the environment, can be removed by cleaning with detergent and water or by disinfection or sterilization.

The degree of cleanliness, that is domestic cleanliness, disinfection or sterilization, will depend on the known or suspected contamination of the equipment and the degree and type of contact with the patient. Equipment should never be shared by patients unless adequate cleaning, disinfection or sterilization can be guaranteed.

Every ambulance carries a wide variety of items of equipment. Some are comparatively simple and in everyday use, whilst others are more complex and less frequently used. All must be properly cared for. Non-disposable equipment of any type is always an infection hazard. It is important to know and understand how to decontaminate and store the equipment to ensure that pathogens are not transferred from one patient to another.

All sterile equipment should be stored in a clean, dry, dust-proof environment.

Disposable items must generally be regarded as such and disposed of after use. The recycling of disposables, if undertaken, requires expert knowledge and must be only undertaken with the full advice and authority of the infection control team.

Table 6 lists common patient equipment carried on ambulances and the type of cleaning, disinfection or sterilization advised.

Table 6. Cleaning/disinfection of ambulance equipment.

Equipment	First method of choice	Accepted alternative
Airways and endotracheal tubes	Disposable	Wash followed by heat disinfection/ sterilization. Store in a clean environment.
Resuscitation equipment	Wash all parts and follow by heat disinfection. (See manufacturers' instructions for temperature.)	Wash followed by disinfection, e.g. hypochlorite 0.1%. Rinse and dry.
Suction equipment—aspirators		
Catheters	Disposable	
Tubing	Disposable	Wash and dry or heat disinfection (weekly).
Suction jar	Empty carefully, wash and dry and follow with heat disinfection.	Empty carefully, wash and dry.
Oxygen tubing	Disposable	Black rubber—wash and dry weekly.
Masks	Disposable	Non-disposable—wash and dry.

Frequency of cleaning, disinfection or sterilization should be after each patient use unless otherwise stated.

All equipment should be dismantled according to manufacturers' instructions.

When washing equipment, a solution of detergent in warm water should be used.

Water left to stagnate in any equipment is liable to become contaminated with potentially pathogenic microorganisms. Green algae have been known to grow in patient equipment with stagnant water reservoirs.

Reusable humidifiers, including those found in baby incubators, should be drained daily and the apparatus disinfected before refilling. Drinking water for patient use should be replenished daily and the container washed and dried before refilling.

Sterile water in sealed bottles should be used for aseptic procedures, e.g. deliveries. Once opened the container and contents become unsterile and any surplus to requirement should be discarded after use.

Laundry

Launderable items such as blankets, pillowcases and stretcher canvases should be laundered when known or suspected to have been in contact with infectious or infested patients and routinely laundered at least weekly. Items should not be sluiced, even when fouled with blood or faeces, but placed into the appropriate coloured plastic bag for foul linen and double-bagged before sending to the laundry. Used and foul linen should not be handled for counting or any other purposes once it has been placed into laundry bags.

The disposal of waste and handling of used linen

Used laundry and waste require special handling and disposal. All ambulance services should have an organized policy with clear instructions issued to personnel. The policy should be in line with the laundry facilities used by the service.

The health and safety guidelines for the safe disposal of clinical waste issued by the Health and Safety Commission Health Services Advisory Committee, 1982 (available from HMSO) categorize clinical waste into five groups. The document not only gives guidance on the segregation, storage and disposal of waste but also on suitable receptacles, and gives recommendations on colour coding.

Protective clothing

The function of protective clothing is to prevent the contamination of uniform and hands by acting as a barrier to the transfer of microorganisms from the infected host to the carer. Contamination may occur by direct contact with the patient's skin or by contact with bedding, equipment and body excretions. The actual type of protective clothing depends upon the degree of potential contamination and the type of infection. Disposable plastic aprons are the most practical form of protection for the uniform. They are cheap and impermeable to microorganisms and water, quick and simple to put on, and easy to store and dispose of. They protect the front of the uniform which is the area of maximum concentration of contamination. The risk of contaminating the sleeves of the uniform can be reduced by rolling up the sleeves and washing after the apron is removed. Gowns, whilst possibly covering a larger area of the uniform, in fact afford little protection. They are not only permeable to water and moisture but many weaves allow large particles of skin and such debris to pass through.

Masks are generally worn with the intention of preventing the dissemination of microorganisms from the nose and mouth, or protecting the wearer from inhaling air-borne microorganisms disseminated by others. Masks are frequently ill-fitting, uncomfortable and inadequate. They may also lull the wearer into a false sense of security. Studies have shown that there is little value in wearing masks except perhaps for certain high-risk situations in hospital, e.g. nursing major burns or working in the operating theatre. In air-borne spread infections which include spread by droplets and discharges from the nose and throat, e.g. diphtheria and acute tonsillitis, ambulance personnel should try to avoid direct contact by averting their head if a patient coughs or sneezes.

Gloves

Disposable plastic gloves, like aprons, are relatively inexpensive, quick and easy to put on and impermeable to water, and can provide an adequate barrier against known incidence of contamination. Non-sterile gloves should be worn when there is a risk of contamination from faeces, e.g. lifting patients with diarrhoea, or when there is a possible risk of gross contamination by blood that is known or suspected to be positive for hepatitis B antigen or human immunodeficiency virus.

Sterile disposable gloves should be donned prior to an emergency aseptic procedure, e.g. a delivery.

Hands

The spread of infection by direct contact is probably the most important method of transmission. Since the hands cannot be sterilized in the same way as an inanimate object and because the hands are most frequently in direct contact with the contaminated source, they are often implicated as an ideal vehicle for the spread of infection.

Hand washing is therefore one of the most important factors in controlling the incidence of cross-infection. Hand washing should be carried out after any patient has been transported. For most instance an efficient hand wash using an unmedicated soap will suffice. Hands should be thoroughly lathered and vigorously washed for approximately 10 seconds, rinsed and dried thoroughly.

Alternatively, alcohol hand rubs may be used if the hands are physically clean. This is quicker than conventional methods and convenient to use when hand washing facilities are not available, e.g. when setting up an emergency intravenous drip or prior to putting on sterile gloves for an emergency delivery. The use of an alcohol hand rub preparation results in a marked reduction of the bacterial flora and, if properly applied, is more efficient than plain soap and water and equally as efficient as a medicated soap solution. The alcohol preparation should be applied to all surfaces of the hands and rubbed vigorously until they are dry.

There are a number of commercially prepared alcohol rub preparations on the market, either in the form of a liquid or gel or an alcohol-saturated disposable cloth. The liquid and gel contain lanolin to prevent drying of the hands and most contain 0.5% chlorhexidine for added bacteriocidal effect. Isopropyl or ethanol are recommended, provided that the product contains between 40 and 80% alcohol.

Accidental contamination

Blood and other body fluids should always be regarded as a potential source of infection. However, for cross-infection to occur from these sources the blood or body fluid has to gain access to the carer, usually via inoculation, i.e. accidental injection by a used syringe containing blood or via a cut/abrasion of the skin or a bite. When an accidental inoculation of blood or other body fluid has occurred through a wound, bleeding should be encouraged and the area washed with copious amounts of water as soon as possible. The incident should be reported to the doctor in charge of the patient who will, if necessary, carry out the required tests and inform the occupational health department if the patient is positive to a blood-borne disease, such as human immunodeficiency virus. If hepatitis B immunoglobulin is required it must be given within 48 hours of injury. The accident procedure of the employing authority will have to be carried out. When accidental contamination of the mucous membranes occurs via the mouth or nose or via gross contamination of the skin, they should be irrigated with copious amounts of water and the incident should be reported as above. Minor splashes of blood and other fluids on intact skin probably pose little risk but should be washed thoroughly as soon as possible.

Infestation by insects and mites

Fleas (*Pulex irritans—Ctenocephalides*). Fleas are small, wingless insects. Infestation is usually by the cat or dog flea, which greatly outnumber human fleas.

Fleas are able to survive for long periods in the environment without feeding. Survival has been known to be a year or more in cool conditions.

Transmission
This is by close contact, when the flea 'leaps' onto the host.

Protection and control
One or two fleas may sometimes be acquired by ambulance

personnel when transferring patients or visiting their homes. This may be unpleasant, but it is not serious. It is unlikely that infestation of the ambulance will occur, provided that the interior of the ambulance is kept clean, that bedding is changed regularly and that personnel maintain a high level of personal hygiene.

However, if personnel know that they are visiting a house which is likely to be heavily infested with fleas, there are two simple precautions worth taking. Firstly, trouser bottoms can be tucked into socks. Secondly, repellents, e.g. dimethyl phthalate, can be applied to the clothing around the socks, trouser ends, shirt cuffs and neck bands. Fleas need to bypass these areas to reach the host's skin.

Bedding should be sent to the laundry immediately after transporting patients known or suspected to be infested with fleas. No special precautions need to be taken with the bedding other than transporting them in the appropriate colour-coded bag.

Mites (*Sarcoptes scabiei*). Infestation with this mite (sarcoptic itch or acariasis) results in scabies. A small mite, the mature female burrows under the host's skin, remaining there for the rest of her life, approximately 30 days, whilst laying eggs. Following invasion, scabies mites quickly multiply in the skin. Irritation usually begins slowly, developing after 6–8 weeks in persons who have not previously been infested.

Transmission
The scabies mite cannot jump from one person to another but has to crawl. Spread is usually by prolonged skin contact with the infested host.

Protection and control
No special protective clothing need be worn. Ambulance personnel having had skin contact with known or suspected cases of scabies should wash their hands and arms after handling the patient. Any skin rash or irritation occurring in the following 3–8 weeks should be reported.

Clothing and bedding are of no importance in scabies transmission as the mite soon dies once off the human body.

Lice. There are three types of human louse: the head louse, the crab louse and the body louse. All are specific to man and each is specific to particular areas of the body.

The head louse (Pediculus capitis)

This is a very small insect which prefers to live its entire life of approximately 35–40 days on the head of its host. The only time that a healthy louse leaves the host's head is to transfer onto another head. Lice found on clothing or bedding are either dead or dying.

Transmission
Head lice do not jump or fly but crawl from one head to another by direct transfer or hair-to-hair contact.

Protection and control
Head-to-head contact should be avoided. When lifting and carrying patients this is not always possible and from time to time ambulance personnel will acquire head lice.

Treatment should be as prompt as possible and should include all close family contacts. Itching and irritation may take 8–10 weeks to develop. People may be quite unaware of the presence of head lice during this time. By the time they are noticed lice may well have been passed onto others.

The local pharmacist will give guidance in respect of which insecticide to use. Some local health authorities operate an insecticide rotation programme in an attempt to reduce the problems related to resistance developed by the lice.

Clothing and bed linen present no risk and no special precautions need to be taken.

The crab louse (Phthirus pubis)

These are commonly found on any hairy part of the body below the neckline. However, they may also be found in the margins of the scalp, particularly in persons with sparse hair, and occasionally in eyelids, eyebrows, beards and moustaches.

Transmission. Crab lice, like other lice, do not jump or fly but crawl from one body to another by direct hair-to-hair contact. Transmission is therefore normally by close body contact.

Protection and control. There is very little risk of ambulance personnel acquiring crab lice whilst transporting patients. Clothing and bedding pose very little risk as the crab louse soon starves to death once off the host. Bedding should be laundered after contact with known or suspected cases of crab lice; no special laundry precautions are needed.

The clothing louse or body louse (Pediculus humanus corporis)

Clothing lice spend most of their lives on the fibres of clothing in much the same way that head lice live on hair. The lice normally prefer the inside of undergarments next to the skin where it is warm. It is a rare event to see lice on the outside of clothing. When the host's body is relaxed and quiet, the lice feed. They may wander about the seams of clothing for some considerable distance.

Transmission. Transmission may be by direct contact with the infested person or indirectly by contact with their clothing.

Protection and control. The lice have a strong dislike for bright light and as a rule do not move far under such conditions. When lifting patients known or suspected of being infested with clothing lice, there are few practical precautions that can be taken. Sleeves should be rolled up and work undertaken in as much light as possible. The lice will thereby be discouraged from moving and will find it hard to hide in the seams of the uniform.

All clothing and bedding suspected of being infested should be turned inside out and treated in a tumble dryer at a temperature of 60°C for 15 minutes or 50°C for 30–35 minutes in order to destroy the crab lice. After the heat treatment laundering may proceed in the normal manner.

10

Control and Communications

The ambulance service has advanced considerably in the field of control and communications to a stage where existing new technology is being introduced to plan and control patient movements in both the emergency and outpatient controls.

Ambulance personnel should realize that if they wish to advance through the rank structure with career objectives set for senior management or above, they must have an appreciation and working knowledge of this most important branch of the service.

This chapter lays out principles, concepts, rules and objectives that should enable ambulance personnel to advance their knowledge, and acts as terms of reference in any future courses or working environment.

THE NATIONAL HEALTH SERVICE ACT, 1977

This act places a duty on the Secretary of State to provide ambulance services 'to such extent as he considers necessary to meet all reasonable requirements'. Guidance to health authorities on what services they should provide on behalf of the Secretary of State is given in DHSS Circular HS(78)45.

The NHS Patient Transport Services Working Party said that 'the NHS should provide or arrange the provision of suitable transport free of charge for:

- Patients requiring transport to hospital as a result of accident, emergency or serious illness
- Patients who suffer from a physical or mental illness, disability or condition who, in the opinion of a doctor (or other authorized health care professional), would be precluded from making their own way to or from necessary treatment or diagnosis without such transport'

The principal function of an ambulance control is to coordinate and comply with the legitimate demands made upon the service and to ensure the optimum use of resources to the benefit of patients.

The following groups can make demands upon the service:

- The public (emergency calls)
- Hospitals, at the instance of doctors
- General practitioners, dentists and midwives

In an emergency anyone can dial '999' and request help from the service. The caller is routed through the British Telecom (BT) exchange to an ambulance emergency control centre, where the caller is put in direct contact with control staff who, having been given the details of the case, can respond by sending the appropriate resource to the incident.

Other requests for non-emergency patients usually have to give 24–48 hours notice, although provision has to be made for the receipt of urgent late treatment/appointment bookings.

Ambulance controls can either be emergency and non-emergency combined, as in some county services, or, as in large metropolitan areas, centralized controls responsible for emergency cover, with corresponding sub/divisional controls to handle the non-emergency work.

Whether a single tier or two-tier service, the roles of those planning and controlling are the same, as follows:

- To receive requests from the public, other emergency services, hospitals, GPs and other health care professionals
- To analyse the details of each request and determine their priority
- To allocate the appropriate resource to meet the demand
- To evaluate response performance

THE RECEIPT OF CALLS

Requests are usually received by control assistants over the telephone and data is recorded using forms AS1 and AS2. Form AS1 is used for emergency incidents. Form AS2 is a request for ambulance transport for a non-emergency journey. Most ambulance authorities use a back-up of tape-recording to monitor conversations for any future enquiry.

While the call is being accepted, consideration has to be given to the difficulties of language barriers, poor telephone reception, distressed relatives or others, incorrect information and the complexities of topography. Control assistants are trained in these fields but always have a more senior rank to whom they can refer.

Most ambulance requests for advance outpatient bookings are sent by the hospitals either by post or, in some cases, by a system of collection. There are still many calls 'phoned in' by the hospital booking clerks, especially where short-notice appointments are concerned.

THE INFORMATION COLLECTED ON FORM AS1

- Date
- Caller's name, address and telephone number
- Location and nature of the incident
- Number of casualties
- Other hazards (fire) and whether anyone is trapped
- Time call is taken and by whom
- Activation time
- Vehicle sent and by whom
- Time at the scene of the incident
- Time at which the service left the scene
- Time of arrival at the hospital and the hospital's name
- Time at which the ambulance was ready for the next job
- Patient's name, address and suspected injuries
- Others notified (police, fire brigade, etc.), when and by whom

In the case of patients taken ill suddenly at home:

- Whether the patient is in bed
- Whether a doctor has been called and, if so, when
- The doctor's name and telephone number
- The doctor's instructions
- By whom the call was taken and when it was received

THE INFORMATION COLLECTED ON FORM AS2

- Patient's name
- Whether they will be accompanied by an escort
- Address they will travel from and to
- Date and time of appointment
- Mobility of the patient (stretcher? walker? double hand?)
- Reason for travel (outpatient? day hospital? remedial?)
- Admission, transfer or discharge?
- By whom the transport was requested
- Doctor authorizing the journey, date, time and telephone number
- Any special instructions
- When and by whom the request was received

PRIORITY AND ANALYSIS OF CALLS

Decisions in the above field are made by control officers. They make their decisions on two main factors:

- The priority of the call
- The ambulance resource available at the time

Calls in are placed in four categories:

- Emergency
- Urgent
- Special
- Planned

Emergency

Calls with this priority must be dealt with immediately, even if other work is delayed or cancelled, e.g.:

- All accident and sudden illness patients
- Maternity patients, unless a clear indication of a time delay is given
- Any other patients for whom emergency procedure is necessary

Urgent

This phrase is used when a definite time limit is imposed and includes such calls as:

- Maternity patients not given emergency priority
- Hospital admissions for which the doctor has given a specified time, e.g. within 1 hour

The word URGENT must always be followed by the time limit for the patient to arrive at the hospital.

Special

This form is used when punctuality is of special importance, e.g.:

- Special treatment, haemodialysis, radio therapy
- Patients to be taken to, or met from, trains, aircraft or boats

Planned

This category comprises those patients not classified in the above three categories, i.e. the majority of outpatients.

Although this priority is lower than the others, punctuality in meeting appointments and minimum waiting times after treatment are important.

THE ALLOCATION OF AMBULANCES

In the emergency and urgent situation, the control officer has to base his decisions on the number of calls to which he has already responded and the availability of ambulance resources to meet the incoming demand. At certain busy periods of the day the stress and responsibility of these decisions can be very demanding. If the control officer meets the situation of having to respond to an emergency/urgent call but has no resources to allocate, he has a problem. There are a number of options he can take:

- Call a neighbouring authority or division to assist, although this may cause a delay in arrival.
- Call an emergency vehicle that has already responded to an earlier emergency of lower priority to assess and report back, where a delay would not unduly affect his patient. They could possibly give ambulance aid until a vehicle could be despatched.
- Call any available officer of the service to respond and give immediate first aid.
- If there is a regional/area training centre then this facility would perhaps be available to send vehicles/staff to the incident.
- The police or fire brigade could be asked to respond and give immediate first aid until resources allow for a vehicle to be despatched.

In the case of major emergency, all authorities have contingency plans within the control rooms to instigate in such an event.

COMPUTERS

Many controls are developing and currently operating computerized planning systems to assist in the production of planned schedules and statistical information which can assist those responsible for the ordering of transport and the costs involved.

Computers are also being developed within emergency controls to assist officers in their decision making. These real-time command systems are expensive and the software (programs) is yet to be developed, although a number of computer organizations are working towards this aim.

There are basically two types of computerized planning systems currently in operation within outpatient controls:

- **A preferred route system** where patient information is input and the preferred vehicle route journeys are established by the planning officer. This system seems to work reasonably well for county areas but does not meet the demands of large metropolitan cities.

- **A fully automatic manning/scheduling system** that plans mathematically using set parameters. Such a system is proving to be a valuable tool in assisting control staff in the day-to-day planning/scheduling of patient journeys with the production of statistics and costs for the district health authorities.

Computer hardware and software

Hardware is the actual machine, which is a box of electronics. There are micro, mini and mainframe computers. Mainframes are large-memory computers capable of holding and processing large amounts of data. They are, of course, very expensive; you could talk in figures of millions of pounds. The microcomputer is known as the home computer, although over the last few years it has become very powerful with the development of the microchip. The minicomputer seems to be the machine of choice and cost. It can support multi-user networks and it can use high level language systems. These operating systems are software programs built in by the manufacturers. It also allows programmers to write in high-level language software programs, e.g. Pascal, 'C' and Fortran. The facility also exists to back up all data that is input onto magnetic tape. In the event of hardware, software or electrical failure, the data is not lost and can be restored into the machine once the fault has been rectified.

It is not necessary for ambulance staff to learn how to programme computers. Specialist help is always available from both the hardware and software suppliers to assist in implementation and in the training of staff.

Computer data input

Basically a computerized planning system requires the following five files of data to be input into its memory banks by ambulance control staff:

Patient data file. A 'menu' appears on the visual display screen (VDU) in a similar fashion to an AS2 form. Details about the patient are typed in the appropriate fields by control assistants (Fig. 10.1). For example:

- Name of patient
- Mobility, address from, address to
- Clinic attending, appointment time
- Days of travel, start date, finish date
- Date of input, time and by whom
- Name of those ordering and telephone number
- Any escorts, priority field (which tells the computer whether to place the patient in the general plan or to designate to a pre-

```
C.I.T 1.1££££££££££££££££££££PATIENT REGISTRATION££££££££££££££££££££££££DD:MM:YY
: PATIENT NAME  [                        ]      MOBILITY  [ ]                    :
: COLLECT FROM  [                                                            ]  :
:               [                                                            ]  :
:                                                                               :
: DELIVER TO    [                                                            ]  :
:               [                                                            ]  :
: HOSP/CLINIC   [     ]/[                        ]         APPT TIME  [      ]  :
:                 mtwtfss                                                        :
: DAYS OF TRAVEL [       ]        RECEIVED DATE [      ] TIME [     ] BY [    ] :
: FIRST VISIT    [      ]         REQ BY [                    ] [            ]  :
: LAST VISIT/UFN [      ]         ESCORTS [ ]   PRIORITY [ ]     CHARGE [ ]     :
: AOI [                                                  ][    ][         ]     :
:                                                                               :
££££££££££££££££££££££££££££££££££££££££££££££££££££££££££££££££££££££££££££££££££
```

Fig. 10.1   VDU display for patient data input.

allocated field vehicle or even to ignore completely so that it
can be planned manually as in the case of a very important
appointment)
• Information field. Anything typed in this field can be printed
on the driver's sheet.

There are also fields to update details about the patient on the
day of travel, e.g. no removals, cancellations/amendments, late
bookings and after-treatments.

Hospital clinic file.   This is a file of individual clinics. Information
is typed in regarding districts, hospitals, the clinic name and the
speciality or type of clinic (Fig. 10.2).
For example:

0 is a remedial clinic
1 is a day hospital clinic
2 is an outpatient clinic
3 is an admission clinic
4 is a discharge clinic
5 is a day surgery clinic
6 is a transfer clinic

recording the throughput time, the earliest opening time of the
clinic and the latest arrival time.

```
C.I.T 1.1££££££££££££££££CLINIC ALTERATION AND DISPLAY£££££££££££££££££DD:MM:YY
:            HEALTH DISTRICT  [                    ]                           :
:    HOSPITAL NAME/MNEMONIC  [                ]/[    ]                         :
:       CLINIC NAME/MNEMONIC  [                    ]/[          ]              :
:     CONSULTANT/SPECIALTY  [                      ]/[                    ]    :
:                            mtwtfss                                          :
:               DAY OF WEEK  [       ]                                        :
:               CLINIC TYPE  [ ]                                              :
:     THROUGHPUT/RETURN TIME  [     ]                                         :
:       ARRIVAL/PICK-UP TIME  -       EARLIEST [   ]    LATEST  [   ]         :
:       ARRIVAL PUNCTUALITY  -        EARLY  [   ]      LATE  [   ]           :
:       RETURN PUNCTUALITY  -         EARLY  [   ]      LATE  [   ]           :
:                              Next/Previous/Alter/Delete  ? [ ]             :
£££££££££££££££££££££££££££££££££££££££££££££££££££££££££££££££££££££££££££££££
```

Fig. 10.2   VDU display for hospital data input.

For example:
- Throughput time for the average remedial clinic in the outpatient department is 90 minutes
- Earliest opening time—0900 hours; latest arrival—1700 hours
- Arrive early—40 minutes; arrive late—40 minutes
- Earliest pick-up—0 minutes; latest pick-up—60 minutes

Street index file.   This is a file of all the addresses within the area served, and in the case of a metropolitan area can be up to over 30 000 streets. When a patient's address or destination is typed in, the computer checks the address details with the street file, and if it does not match, which it must do letter for letter, then it will not accept the version typed in by the control assistant and will alert the control assistant by placing a flashing pointer (cursor) at the start of the address they typed in (Fig. 10.3).

Vehicle file.   The planning officer receives from the ambulance stations his daily allocation of vehicle resource and manning levels. His task is to type in this information on a visual display menu for the day he is planning (Fig. 10.4). The menu displays:

- A vehicle call sign and a classification of the vehicle, e.g. Class 1 vehicles are recognized by the computer as two-man vehicles

```
C.I.T 1.1££££££££££££££££££££££££££ADDRESS ENTRY£££££££££££££££££££££££££££DD:MM:YY
:                              ADDRESS PART                              ZONE    :
: 1: [                                                        ]      [   ]       :
:                                                                               :
: 2: [                                                        ]      [   ]       :
:                                                                               :
: 3: [                                                        ]      [   ]       :
:                                                                               :
: 4: [                                                        ]      [   ]       :
:                                                                               :
: 5: [                                                        ]      [   ]       :
:                                                                               :
: 6: [                                                        ]      [   ]       :
:                                                                               :
: 7: [                                                        ]      [   ]       :
:                                                                               :
: 8: [                                                        ]      [   ]       :
:                                                                               :
: 9: [                                                        ]      [   ]       :
:                                                                               :
:10: [                                                        ]      [   ]       :
££££££££££££££££££££££££££££££££££££££££££££££££££££££££££££££££££££££££££££££££££
```

Fig. 10.3 VDU display for entry of patients' addresses.

```
C.I.T 1.1£££££££££££££££££££££££VEHICLE DETAILS ENTRY££££££££££££££££££££££££££DD:MM:YY
:                                                                               :
:   CALL SIGN [        ]      CLASS [ ]   BASE [  ]     SEATS [ ]                :
:                                                                               :
:                     mtwtfss                                                   :
:   DAYS AVAILABLE    [      ]          SHIFT - START [   ]  END [   ]           :
:         STATUS      [ ]               BREAK - START [   ]  END [   ]           :
:         AREAS       [  ][  ][  ][  ][  ]                                       :
:                                                                               :
:   CAR SERVICE :    NAME [              ]        PHONE [       ]                :
:                                                                               :
:                                                                               :
££££££££££££££££££££££££££££££££££££££££££££££££££££££££££££££££££££££££££££££££££
```

Fig. 10.4 VDU display for entry of vehicle details.

capable of carrying all mobilities, Class 8 perhaps as one-man vehicles (solos), Class 14 as taxi vehicles.
- The seating capacity.
- The starting point. This is represented by a zone number which is an address from where the vehicle starts and corresponds to the street file and travel time matrix file.
- A status classification field. For example, if 'P' is typed into the menu, then the vehicle will be used by the computer in the general plan and a whole day's work will be allocated to this vehicle. 'A' typed in means that the vehicle will not be given any patients but will be made available for the planning officer to create a journey for specific patients. 'PV' typed in would tell the computer to allocate only those patients whose code in the priority field of the patient data file are to be placed on this vehicle, usually pre-allocated day hospital patients.

The planning officer will also type in the shift start and finish, the time of the lunch break, and special zone numbers to perhaps restrict vehicle movement to certain areas or hospitals.

Travel matrix file.   This file contains all the travel and handling times from zone to zone within the area served. This is a very large file containing up to 300 000 travel times.

The patient data and vehicle files are everyday tasks to be input into the computer. The hospital clinic, street index and travel matrix files, once created, only need occasional updates.

The average outpatient control dealing with 1500–2000 patient journeys a day will need at least three fast C/As typing AS2 data all day to enable the planning officers to plan.

The computer plan

The planning officer inputs the day's date of travel and asks the computer to generate a plan. The computer then calls all the patients for that date of travel and allocates them to the available vehicles. Any patients, due to clinic parameter or travel constraints, that the computer cannot plan are displayed on an unallocated list. This can either be on the VDU screen or printed onto hard copy.

The planning officers have the option to view all journeys and to alter or amend whatever they are not in agreement with. For example, they can delete a patient from a journey, move a patient from one journey to another, insert a patient from the unallocated list onto a journey, change start and finish times of vehicles, create a journey for a vehicle and insert patients onto that journey. Many other options are available to the planners to optimize the best plan.

The parameter file

There is also a plan parameter file which influences the way the computer plans. These parameters allow vehicles to only do certain things and it is careful analysis and adjustment of these times and figures which produces the best plan (Fig. 10.5). For example, one of the parameters is called 'dead time' or 'travel empty time'. This is the amount of time a vehicle is allowed to run empty to its first pick-up—say 20 minutes. If you have a low dead time, patients will not be picked up and therefore not included in the plan. If you have a high dead time, vehicles are underproductive and the same result will occur.

```
C.I.T 1.1ƐƐƐƐƐƐƐƐƐƐƐƐƐƐƐƐƐƐƐƐƐƐPLAN PARAMETERSƐƐƐƐƐƐƐƐƐƐƐƐƐƐƐƐƐƐƐƐƐƐƐƐƐDD:MM:YY
:                                                                            :
:              DEAD TIME  [   ]                                              :
:                                                                            :
:           NEAR TO BASE  [   ]                                              :
:                                                                            :
:      DETOUR MULTIPLIER  [   ]                                              :
:                                                                            :
:        DETOUR MAXIMUM   [   ]                                              :
:                                                                            :
:     MILEAGE CONVERSION  [   ]/[   ]                                        :
:                                                                            :
:                ORDER    [                                                  ]
:                                                                            :
:  ENFORCED BREAKS (y/n)? [ ]                                                :
:  ENFORCED EARLY  (y/n)? [ ]                                                :
:                                                                            :
:   TRAVEL TIME ADJUSTER  [   ]                                              :
:                                                                            :
:   HOSPITAL NEAR FACTOR  [   ]                                              :
:                                                                            :
:      DIRECTION FACTOR   [   ]                                              :
:                                                         print required? [ ]:
ƐƐƐƐƐƐƐƐƐƐƐƐƐƐƐƐƐƐƐƐƐƐƐƐƐƐƐƐƐƐƐƐƐƐƐƐƐƐƐƐƐƐƐƐƐƐƐƐƐƐƐƐƐƐƐƐƐƐƐƐƐƐƐƐƐƐƐƐƐƐƐƐƐƐƐƐ
```

Fig. 10.5 VDU display for parameter input.

Computerized planning is still in its infancy, although ambulance services must advance with positive forward-looking strategies towards the fulfilment of this technological field. Do not fear computers—learn and read about them—they are only an aid to the human brain and will only fail if those that operate them do not follow the rules and procedures in the application of data input.

MANUAL PLANNING: OUTPATIENT CONTROL

There must always be procedures in the event of computer failure. Normally, as previously mentioned, a control system manager will have most of his data, e.g. patient details, backed up on magnetic tape and can reload this information when the software or hardware faults are rectified. The problem is time. Can the fault be rectified in time to produce the schedules? A decision must be made which may mean working very late or even planning manually. It must always be possible to plan manually from AS2 information. If patient AS2 data is input directly from hospitals, and the computer system has a major malfunction in its hardware or electrical supply, then a plan could not be achieved, resulting in patient cancellations.

Outpatient appointments fall into two categories:

- Regulars, e.g. patients who travel everyday or two or three times a week
- One-offs, e.g. consultant and outpatient appointments

When a planning officer plans manually he will usually follow the following procedures, or a similar format:

- Select AS2s for the day's travel.
- Check for any late cancellations or amendments.
- Check the dates of travel—there may be misfiled dates included.
- Look for OBs (outside boundaries). Most authorities have a coordinating officer who will be in touch with other services that may be in your area and who can help by taking your patient in the return journey or vice versa.
- Sort the AS2s into appointment times, e.g. 0900–1000–1100 hours.
- Sort the AS2s according to the patients' mobility (stretcher, walker, double hand). Look for any special instructions, e.g. must travel alone, walk out, lie down, oxygen required.
- Sort the AS2s into pick-up areas, usually by zones.
- Analyse the patient destinations, i.e. the hospital and unit they are attending.
- Analyse the manning levels and vehicle resource.
- Build runs and loads according to priority, e.g. radio therapy—dialysis and computed axial tomography scans take priority over physiotherapy and outpatient appointments.
- When loads are built up and put into runs, C/As can type out schedules.
- The planning officer will draw up a schedule plan displaying who will be doing what, where and when.

Some vehicles should be left spare in case of sickness, late bookings and after-treatments or vehicle breakdowns.

DIFFICULTIES IN CONTROL

Controlling a fleet of 50 or more vehicles not only requires skill by the duty officer in charge but also team-work of those assisting him, which includes ambulance personnel.

As previously mentioned, computer technology is being introduced and developed as an aid to decision making. Some controls have computers in the emergency side that will tell a controller the nearest first and second vehicle response. There are radio systems that alert the controller as to vehicle availability or whether they are on the way to or from an incident. Street maps, indexes and clerical information can be stored and made available at the touch of a button.

The emergency controller's main asset is that he always has a minimum manning level which, if it drops due to sickness or other reasons, is replaced from other sources, e.g. the non-emergency crews. When all his emergency crews are engaged, again he can call on non-emergency vehicles to respond. Obviously, things can get very hectic and he has a great responsibility to respond vehicles within the operational research consultants' (Orcon) standards. It must be appreciated that the press and the public are very quick in complaining about any delay.

One problem with two-tier services is that the emergency controller only knows the state of availability of his emergency vehicles. When he is busy and under pressure he may respond with a vehicle that comes or is clear from some distance away from the incident, whereas there may have been a nearer non-emergency vehicle available or even engaged, but close to the incident, that could at least have responded and given ambulance aid. Patients and the public do not really mind what vehicle arrives as long as assistance can be given and help is on the way; what they do not accept is a long delay. Emergency controllers obviously get in touch with outpatient controls and ask for assistance, but this can cause a time delay. What they need is direct access to divisional outpatient control's radio channels and to relay a priority call for any vehicle within the vicinity.

Real-time computers of the command system type used by the police would enable emergency controllers to know at all times the state and availability of all vehicles.

The number of incidents to which an emergency control responds can be unpredictable. Manning levels are developed over the years by analysis of averages, and on balance work out reasonably well; on the other hand, non-emergency outpatient controls have daily fixed patient journey targets to achieve. Obviously, if you have planned 1500–2000 patient journeys then you need the required manning levels and vehicles to deliver the service. If any of these resources are removed, either to the emergency side or as a result of sickness, the outpatient controller may have to cancel patients according to priority, or try to slot them in onto other vehicles which will cause delays in arrival and departure. It should be remembered that vehicles will be fully planned for the day and unless the controller has access, he has very little flexibility.

Since the new salary structure for ambulance personnel has been introduced, authorities have been able to re-negotiate new 'stand-alone' rotas which have built-in relief, and extended day shifts. This will allow more flexibility in that previously the bulk of ambulance personnel worked from 8 a.m. to 4 p.m. and controllers relied on overtime to get patients home. With the introduction of the new salary structure, which had to be self-financing, overtime is now very limited with a maximum of 2 hours per man per week.

Another difficulty is the provision of lunch-breaks. This is not so much a problem on the emergency side because they can always call a crew off their break to respond to the incident. The problem is on the outpatient side where a break must be taken after no more than $5\frac{1}{2}$ hours of work. A planned day's work gives drivers a break, but when dealing with a large fleet and hundreds of journeys, things go wrong and crews invariably run late. In large metropolitan cities, the traffic conditions, weather, no-removal delays in patients not being ready, wrong addresses, cancelled appointments, etc., can all affect the pick-up and arrival of patients. If patients arrive late then it is around the midday period that they have to go home. This clashes with lunch-breaks and also has a knock-on effect in that you also have to get your 1400–hour appointments in. Patients may well have been planned to be taken home by other vehicles and not by the one that took them in. If they arrive late for their appointments then they will not be ready when vehicles arrive to take them home. They then have to be re-planned manually off the control board. The duty control officer has the responsibility of having to re-allocate these patients, and at the present moment in time has to try and remember with the aid of a very detailed paper schedule where his vehicles are, who is running late, and 50 patients on his unallocated board with appointments to and from 20 or more different hospitals.

PERFORMANCE EVALUATION

Those responsible for the evaluation of performance standards are senior control staff who are accountable to their principal and chief officer for the day-to-day operation of the control function and the production of statistics. They are also responsible for operating within defined budgets, vehicle resource and staff rota levels.

The quality of ambulance services is measured by comparing performance with Orcon standards. There are separate standards for different types of journeys and priorities, and different standards devised for metropolitan and non-metropolitan services. The standards require that in a set proportion of patient journeys, known as the percentile, specified time limits should be kept.

An emergency vehicle with a fully trained crew should be on its way within 3 minutes of receipt of a '999' call 95 times out of 100, and the vehicle should reach the patient within 14 minutes for metropolitan services or within 20 minutes for non-metropolitan services.

Other information that managers need to monitor concerning the quality of service and the efficiency of the use of resources are:

- Totals of patients' journeys—mileage and cost
- Cost per patient journey
- Cost per vehicle mile
- Miles per patient journey
- Number of patients per vehicle journey
- Vehicle utilization

MOBILE RADIO SYSTEMS

Radio communication systems have advanced dramatically with the introduction of the microchip. Telephone companies and large developers of radio systems can supply almost any system to suit the need of an ambulance authority. Equipment is almost limitless, with only the cost affecting decisions of implementation. The technology of these communication systems is beyond the scope of this chapter. The following paragraphs explain in simple terms the theory and concepts in radio communication that may well be of interest to ambulance personnel.

The development of VHF radio

During the 1939–45 war, the need for communications to aircraft and ships resulted in a radio–telephone system based on short range VHF (very high frequency) radio being developed. The range is very short because radiation at these very high frequencies is largely restricted to semi-optical limitations, i.e. the line of sight.

Immediately after the war, the need for improved communications in the police and fire services resulted in further applications of these wartime developments. This time, the communications were directed towards achieving the passing of messages to and from the drivers of vehicles.

Because of the short range of the VHF system, it was found to be possible to use the same radio channel several times, relying on geographical separation to prevent one user interfering with another. It was realized that this new development could be used

Table 7. The Orcon standards.

Measure of performance	Percentile	Metropolitan services (standard values)	Non-metropolitan services (standard values)
Emergencies			
Activation time	95	3 minutes	3 minutes
Response time	50	7 minutes	8 minutes
	95	14 minutes	20 minutes
Urgent cases			
Arrival time in relation to scheduled arrival time	95	4 minutes late	5 minutes late
Non-emergencies			
Ambulance load to and from treatment centre	50	2 patients	2 patients
	95	8 patients	8 patients
Arrival time in relation to appointment time			
Planned	5	40 minutes early	60 minutes early
	25	20 minutes early	30 minutes early
	75	15 minutes early	20 minutes early
	95	40 minutes early	60 minutes early
Special	5	40 minutes early	60 minutes early
	5	20 minutes early	30 minutes early
	75	10 minutes late	15 minutes late
	95	20 minutes late	30 minutes late
Waiting time after treatment	50	30 minutes	30 minutes
	95	60 minutes	60 minutes

in many other activities, and the post office, which controlled the licensing of private radio systems at that time, made available a number of VHF wavelengths or channels for business use and other activities.

The new tool was speedily adopted by hire cars, taxis, ambulances, electricity and water authorities, doctors, vets, tugs, other small craft and a host of other users. On a historical note, the very first private radio licences issued in this country were for a fleet of tugs in the Tyne and Wear rivers and for a fleet of 'Camtax' radio taxis in Cambridge in 1947.

The principles of carrier waves and modulation systems

A radio transmitter is simply a generator of high-frequency alternating current. This current is fed into an aerial system so that the current oscillates up and down the aerial at the prescribed frequency to which the transmitter is tuned. The energy in the aerial produces a fluctuating electromagnetic field, which leaves the aerial in the form of electromagnetic waves, and is known as the carrier wave.

It is necessary to arrange for this same carrier wave to carry some speech intelligence. In the first instance the voice produces a sound wave, and a microphone is used to convert this sound energy into its equivalent in electrical energy known as the 'audio wave'. The audio wave is superimposed on the carrier wave to produce either an amplitude-modulated (AM) carrier or a frequency-modulated (FM) carrier.

In the case of amplitude modulation the carrier wave from a transmitter has had the *amplitude* (i.e. height) of the carrier wave form altered in sympathy with the audio wave, while in the case of frequency modulation the carrier wave has had the actual *frequency* of the carrier wave slightly altered (from its original precise value) in sympathy with the audio wave. By design, the carrier in frequency modulation is not permitted to deviate very far from its basic frequency, not only to prevent the transmitter from drifting into the next wireless channel and causing interference, but also to ensure that it is at the same frequency as the distant receivers, which are to pick up these signals.

Radio receivers are connected to an aerial of critical length tuned to receive a specific carrier frequency. A section of the receiver is designed to detect the modulations on the carrier wave and thus separate or filter the audio wave from the carrier signal. This audio wave is amplified and fed to the loudspeaker, where it is reproduced as the original soundwave once again.

The single-frequency simplex

This is very technical sounding terminology for a very simple arrangement. It merely tells one that a single frequency is used to both transmit and receive, and that a two-way simultaneous communication is not possible. Because of the poor control that can be exercised over the system, it is seldom used. A prime application is perhaps in the case of hand-held portable sets, giving limited range.

The two-frequency simplex

This is the system that is commonly used by most mobile radio systems. The mobiles will use a certain frequency for transmission and another frequency for reception. The control point will have the reciprocal arrangement of these frequencies for transmission and reception. The term 'simplex' advises us that simultaneous two-way transmissions are not possible.

The two-frequency scheme permits the use of what is called 'talk-through' working, whereby any signals received at 'Control' from a mobile are automatically re-transmitted on the 'Control'-transmit frequency. In this manner all mobiles will hear the messages that any mobile is transmitting to 'Control'. This talk-through facility is normally only available on request from a mobile, when 'Control' will switch on the facility for a specific period.

It is worth mentioning here that 'two-frequency talk-through working' considerably increases the working range when compared with the working range of two mobiles using a single frequency scheme.

UHF radio schemes

The use of ultra high frequency (UHF) schemes has certain advantages:

- A short stub aerial—ideal for personal pocket radio
- A short line of sight range—ideal for police divisional radio schemes
- A bounce factor—provides good penetration into buildings

Because of these properties, UHF is commonly used by the emergency services for two-way pocket radio communication. If the UHF pocket radio users wish to communicate with the VHF main control, a UHF/VHF repeater can be installed in a mobile. This piece of equipment, as the name suggests, allows a UHF communication to be repeated to the VHF control on the VHF frequency.

'Mute' or 'squelch' controls

All mobiles on early mobile radio systems had to suffer continual background 'mush' or interference on the loudspeakers in their mobiles. This background noise was caused by low level signals such as ignition interference and general extraneous signals.

This sort of interference noise should not be present in the modern mobile radio system by virtue of a mute or squelch control built into the wireless equipment. This mute control is basically a device which maintains the loudspeaker switched off until a signal of a certain strength is received. The adjustment of this critical signal level is sometimes an internal adjustment and sometimes there is an external 'mute' control provided. This level may typically be set at 2 microvolts, and therefore interference signals of less value than 2 microvolts will not 'switch on' the receiver, and as a result the mobile loudspeaker is silent until a recognized signal is received.

Remote bay stations and associated links

It is seldom found that the site for radio control is ideal for 'line of sight' communication to mobiles, and hence it is necessary to position main station equipment at some remote site, generally on a hill or a high building. A radio control point therefore has to utilize a remote control unit which is linked to the hill-top main station either by a BT land line or a radio link.

A BT land line is generally used when the distance from the hill-top site to the control point is not excessive. A single pair of cables can be utilized to provide a speech path and two switching functions by the clever use of centre-tap transformers at each end.

Despite this economy of circuits, if the distance between the 'control' and the hill-top site is considerable, then the BT costs will be prohibitive and a radio link is used. To achieve the latter, however, it is important that a good line-of-sight link is available between the two points. Until recently, a radio link was normally achieved by utilizing two UHF frequencies for 'send' and 'receive'. Shortage of UHF channels has made more common the use of microwave links in mobile systems operating generally in the 1.5 GHz bands, and although the microwave links are more expensive, multiplexing techniques allow one microwave link to carry a large number of channels. At these frequencies, the wavelength is approaching close to that of light waves. It is not surprising then that we can use somewhat similar techniques. Hence an aerial dish is used, which is similar to a searchlight reflector, and this concentrates the energy into a narrow beam so that quite large distances can be covered by using two opposite-facing dishes. Their use is even more restricted to the line of sight here, and the path must be completely clear of any obstructions.

Again, at these frequencies if conventional co-axial feeder cable is used to connect to these dishes, then nearly all the power would be lost within the feeder cable. Instead, a waveguide is used, where the actual electromagnetic waves are directed through a metallic tube rather than a cable.

Multi-bay stations—their problems and some solutions

ASSORT. There are many mobile radio systems which have coverage provided by as many as five hill-top station sites.

Inevitably the areas of coverage of these stations overlap each other in varying degrees. A mobile calling the 'control' is therefore received at several sites at different strength levels, and when all these signals are brought into the loudspeaker of the control room, it results in a very fluttering signal with a lot of background noise. What is needed is an 'automatic system of selection of received transmissions'. Such a device, known as 'ASSORT,' was designed, and samples all the incoming signals from each main station site. It selects the best signal and suppresses all the others; hence the problem is resolved.

Quasi-sync. On multistation systems, problems can also occur in the reverse direction, i.e. from the control room to the mobile. This is again a situation where the mobile is in an overlap area, i.e. where the mobile is receiving the same signals from more than one main station. Until recently it was not possible to accurately control the frequency of the transmitters, and as they drifted apart the various carrier waves 'beat' against each other to produce a 'beat' frequency of a few hundred hertz upwards that produced a whistle sound in the receivers, which could sometimes make the speech unreadable.

Crystal oscillators are now available which can accurately tie down a transmitter to a precise frequency. By accurately holding two or three transmitters to a deliberate frequency difference of a few hertz, the beat note that is produced is also only a few hertz and is not heard because it is not in the audio range. This arrangement is known as 'quasi-sync' working.

Problems can still occur, however, in areas where signal strengths are equal but where the signal path lengths are different and audio distortion can occur. So it is usual to plan these systems by careful location of the transmitters to avoid large areas where the signals overlap.

It is normal practice in such situations to use a combination of ASSORT and quasi-sync. For example, control will call a mobile using quasi-sync; the mobile will respond and the ASSORT equipment will select the nearest main station to that mobile; that particular main station will then 'lock-in' for the rest of the communication for messages either from control or from the mobile.

Tone lock

With the increase in mobile wireless schemes and the resulting shortage of wireless channels, it is becoming almost impossible to acquire a wireless channel that is not already in use by someone who is within range of your own main stations. As a result, control rooms are being continually disturbed by messages from 'foreign' mobiles.

One solution to this problem now commonly being used by the ambulance services is 'tone lock'. This is an arrangement whereby two exclusive tone signals are used as the key to switch on the main station and mobile receivers respectively. A sub-audio tone is transmitted from the ambulance whenever the ambulance is communicating with its control, and this tone maintains the main station receiver in the 'receive' condition. As a result of this tone lock on the receivers, interference from mobiles from another ambulance scheme does not disturb the control. A similar arrangement exists in relation to transmissions to the mobiles, in that mobiles will only receive messages from their own control.

The only time in fact that interference is heard on a tone-lock scheme is on the occasion that a receiver is switched on by a tone-lock message simultaneously with the reception of a message from a foreign mobile. Normally, however, in such circumstances the signal from the 'home' mobile is still quite readable.

Selective calling

This is basically an extension of the tone-lock principle, except that individual mobiles have their own coded tone signal. In this way a mobile is not disturbed by signals sent to other mobiles, and will only receive messages when they are directed to him.

Whenever a mobile has been selectively called, a lamp is illuminated in the mobile so that if the operator was absent from the vehicle at the time of call, the mobile operator is made aware of this fact when he or she returns to the vehicle.

The tones are transmitted from an 'encoder' in the control room. The encoder will normally transmit a sequential number of tones relating to a particular mobile.

Before a mobile transmits a message on this type of system, it is important that the mobile first depresses a 'defeat' button to establish first that no other transmissions are in progress. More sophisticated systems, however, bring up an 'engaged' lamp in the mobile if any other mobile is occupying the scheme, and this largely obviates the need for a 'defeat' button.

Selective calling can also operate in the opposite direction (i.e. mobile to control) if desired. In this instance a call from the mobile can produce a display of the mobile's call sign in the control room to advise control that that particular mobile wishes to communicate.

Paging systems

Paging systems work basically on the same principles as described previously under 'selective calling'. An encoder will be used to trigger the transmission of various tones over a radio system to pocket pager systems. The number of pagers operating on a mobile radio system is limited by the Home Office to the equivalent number of mobiles on the system.

There is, however, virtually no limit to the number of pagers that can be employed on a dedicated paging system, such as the paging system in a hospital. The latter type of system generally employs one of two frequency bands—27.12 megahertz and 31.75 megahertz. Sometimes the system operates from a free radiating aerial on the top of a hospital, or else it may operate on an inductive loop system whereby the hospital premises are surrounded by a perimeter aerial loop. Some of these systems are now quite sophisticated, where the calling telephone extension number is displayed on the pager. Other systems, used in conjunction with certain type telephone exchanges, allow the telephone operators to be completely bypassed in the paging function. A telephone call to an unattended telephone can be arranged to automatically page the missing person. The paged person then moves to the nearest telephone and dials his own telephone extension to receive the waiting call.

Community repeaters

There have no doubt been occasions in the past where there was a requirement for a mobile radio scheme to control perhaps only two mobiles. Normally the cost of main station equipment, etc., made such small schemes an uneconomic proposition. Recently, however, the Home Office has given approval to the setting up of 'community repeaters' by the commercial radio companies, and this arrangement allows the setting up of mobile radio schemes for very little capital outlay.

The arrangement allows up to 16 mobile radio schemes to operate on one wireless channel. The total number of mobiles on the channel would be limited to approximately 100 mobiles. Each radio scheme would have its own tone-lock frequency so that communications from any particular scheme were private and not disturbing other scheme users.

When the radio channel is being used by one scheme, an 'engaged' lamp is illuminated in all other mobiles to warn them of this fact. There is also an automatic time limit on transmissions to prevent one mobile from monopolizing the channel.

Appendix—Law for Ambulance Personnel

It is not possible to set out the differences that exist between the laws of different countries in this appendix. Scottish law differs mostly in its application rather than in its basic tenets. Thus, although the references will not apply to Scottish law, most of the definitions are identical between the systems.

In countries outside the British Isles there will be considerable differences, although the role of ambulance personnel remains the same. It will be necessary to ascertain the equivalent regulations in each country.

English law has developed over hundreds of years and has only recently been consolidated into a 'code'. Much of the law is the result of individual judgements in various courts.

One principle that does tend to run throughout our law is that a person who acts reasonably should not incur the wrath of the law if what he has done is in fact wrong. Therefore, although a man may have broken the law the penalty levied against him will be less severe if his state of mind is innocent.

What follows is a very brief outline of some of the laws that may affect ambulance personnel. It is intended only as a guide and readers who find their interest aroused can research subjects in detail from the many legal textbooks to be found.

The contents of this chapter are only opinion. The decision of a court may take a different view. Therefore, ambulance staff should seek the advice of professional lawyers in cases concerning them.

ROAD TRAFFIC LAW

Definition of an ambulance

An ambulance is a motor vehicle specially designed and constructed (not merely adapted) for carrying as equipment, permanently affixed to the vehicle, equipment used for medical, dental or health

186

purposes and used primarily for the carriage of persons suffering from illness, injury or disability.

Motor Vehicle (Construction and Use) Regulations, 1978

Parking exemptions for ambulances

Ambulances are exempt from the following restrictions on stopping, where to observe the restrictions would hinder the proper use of the vehicle:

Pelican crossings. Stopping within the limits (between the line of studs and the crossing itself) of the pelican crossing (Pelican Pedestrian Crossing Regulations, 1969).

Zebra crossings. Stopping within the limits (between the area indicated by zig-zag markings) of the zebra crossing (Zebra Pedestrian Crossing Regulations, 1971).

Quitting. Leaving a motor vehicle unattended without first switching off the engine. (The requirement to set the handbrake still applies.) [Motor Vehicles (Construction and Use) Regulations, 1978.]

Double white lines. Stopping alongside an area of road controlled by a pattern of double solid or broken white lines (Traffic Signs Regulations and General Directions, 1981).

Night-time parking. Parking on the offside of the road during the hours of darkness [Motor Vehicles (Construction and Use) Regulations, 1978].

Use of ambulances on motorways

The motorway regulations prohibiting:

- Pedestrians on the motorway
- Driving on the hard shoulder
- Driving on the central reservation
- Stopping on any part of the motorway
- Reversing on the motorway
- Restrictions on the use of lanes

do not apply to:

- Ambulances used for emergencies
- Pedestrians dealing with accidents

Motorway Traffic (England and Wales) Regulations, 1982

Driving exemptions for ambulances

Ambulances are exempt from the legal requirements imposed on the drivers of other vehicles in relation to the following:

Hours of driving. Limitations exist as to hours of driving and rest periods [Road Transport, Drivers' Hours and Records Regulations (EEC) 543/69 as amended]. See also Transport Act (1968) Part IV, Domestic Rules—Drivers' Hours.

Blue lamps. Limitations exist as to colours of lights visible from the front and rear of motor vehicles.

Loads. Restrictions exist on the length and width of loads [Motor Vehicles (Construction and Use) Regulations, 1978].

Keep left/right signs. Ambulances are exempt where to observe these signs would cause a hindrance, provided that no danger is caused to other road users (Traffic Signs Regulations and General Directions, 1981).

Loudspeakers. Restrictions on the use of loudspeakers on vehicles (Control of Pollution Act, 1974).

Audible warning devices. Restrictions on the use of two-tone horns, bells and sirens [Motor Vehicle (Construction and Use) Regulations, 1978].

Horns. Restrictions on the use of warning instruments at night or whilst stationary [Motor Vehicles (Construction and Use) Regulations, 1978].

Dark windows. Restrictions on the transparency of vehicle windows. This requirement is only lifted in relation to the windows fitted to the rear of the driver's seat [Motor Vehicles (Construction and Use) Regulations, 1978].

Speed limits. Speed limits do not apply to vehicles used for police, fire brigade or ambulance purposes if to observe those speed limits would hinder the use of the vehicle in carrying out its purposes (Road Traffic Regulation Act, 1967).

Traffic lights. A vehicle used for ambulance purposes may, when being so used, if necessary for its use on that occasion, pass a red traffic light, provided that to do so is not likely to endanger persons moving past a green light, or force other drivers to change speed or course to avoid an accident, or cause danger to any other road user. (Traffic Signs Regulations and General Directions, 1981).

Bus lanes. There is an implied exemption to bus lane restrictions (Road Traffic Regulation Act, 1984).

Road accidents: the legal requirements

If in any case, owing to the presence of a motor vehicle on a road, an accident occurs whereby:

- Personal injury is caused to any person other than the driver of that vehicle
- Damage is caused to any vehicle (not just motor vehicle) other than that vehicle or any trailer drawn by it
- Injury is caused to any animal other than an animal in or on that vehicle or its trailer, or
- Damage is caused to any property fixed to, constructed on, growing in or otherwise forming part of the land on which the road is situated or on the land adjacent to that road

the driver of that vehicle shall **STOP.**

If required to do so by any person having reason to require it, he shall supply his name and address, the name and address of the owner of the vehicle and the registration mark of the vehicle. In the case of an accident involving personal injury he shall produce to any person with reason to require it his certificate of insurance (or acceptable alternative).

If, for any reason, the driver fails to comply with the requirements to produce insurance or to supply details as above he shall report the accident to a police constable or at a police station as soon as is reasonably practicable, but in any case within 24 hours of the occurrence.

Animal.   For the purposes of road accidents, an animal is described as any horse, cattle, ass, mule, sheep, goat or dog.

Road accidents: careless or reckless driving

Road traffic law provides that it shall be an offence for any person to drive a motor vehicle on a road:

- Without due care and attention
- Without reasonable consideration for other road users
- Recklessly

It is not necessary that there should be an accident before a prosecution will be considered. For example, the 'reasonable consideration' offence covers the behaviour of the driver who deliberately drives through a puddle in order to splash a pedestrian or one who uses his vehicle in a manner likely to frighten other road users.

The word 'reasonable' is most important in determining police policy on prosecution and in court decisions. Whilst the driver of a bus, ahead of its schedule, has been prosecuted for driving very slowly and delaying other drivers, the driver of an ambulance, travelling at the same speed to protect his patient, would not be prosecuted.

An error of judgement does not, of itself, constitute careless driving. To misjudge the speed of an approaching vehicle when pulling out of a junction is less likely to be regarded as careless than the same misjudgement when overtaking. Every case is taken on its merits, having regard for the nature of the road, its use and condition, and the amount of traffic on the road or reasonably expected to be on the road at the time.

In emergencies, ambulance personnel may disregard much of the law relating to the use of vehicles on the road. Even in those instances where he does not have exemption, he is likely to be treated leniently if acting in the best interests of his patient. If he is involved in an accident, however, he is of little value to his patient or the service whether or not he becomes liable to prosecution. It is better to travel a little more slowly than to risk not arriving at all.

OFFENCES AGAINST THE PERSON

It is a sad fact that ambulance personnel are assaulted from time to time. It is also a fact that the normal actions of ambulance personnel may consist of an assault. Defences to assault are therefore of some concern to ambulance personnel, as are the varying degrees of assault which are part of the criminal law.

Definitions

Assault. This is any act which constitutes any attempt, offer or threat to use violence or any unlawful force to the person of another.

Battery. This is the actual application of unlawful force to the person of another without his consent.

For an assault to be punishable by the criminal law there must be the intentional or reckless application of unlawful physical force.

Degrees of assault

Common assault. Section 42—Offences Against the Person Act (1861) deals with very minor common law assaults. Police do not normally take action but refer parties to civil redress or private prosecution.

Aggravated assault. Section 43—Offences Against the Person Act (1861) deals with assault on a female or child aggravated by the degree of assault.

Assault occasioning actual bodily harm. Section 47—Offences Against the Person Act (1861) deals with some form of hurt or injury interfering with health or comfort.

Wounding or inflicting grievous bodily harm. Section 20—Offences Against the Person Act (1861)—deals with:

- Wounding—defined as a breaking of the whole skin, allowing blood to flow
- Grievous bodily harm—defined as seriously interfering with normal health or comfort

Wounding or causing grievous bodily harm with intent. Section 18—Offences Against the Person Act (1861) differs from Section 20 by virtue of intent to cause harm or resist arrest.

Defences to a charge of assault

- Accident—if carrying out a lawful act with reasonable care
- Consent—if consent, to a lawful act, is given freely by a rational and sober person
- Lawful correction—by parent, guardian or teacher
- Defence of family or servant
- Execution of legal or official duty
- Defence of one's property

Section 3 Criminal Law Act (1967). A person may use such force as is reasonable in the circumstances in the prevention of crime or in effecting or assisting in the lawful arrest of offenders or suspected offenders or of persons unlawfully at large.

Many of these defences are self-explanatory. The particular application to the ambulance service is in two parts:

- When ambulance personnel are assaulted they are entitled to defend themselves. They may only use whatever force is reasonable to do so.
- Many of the acts carried out by ambulance personnel in carrying out their duty may be assaults. It is a defence that a lawful act was carried out with reasonable care.

Homicide

Homicide is the lawful or unlawful killing of a human being by a human being. It can therefore be either criminal or non-criminal.

Non-criminal homicide

- Lawful execution
- Accident—where a person kills another whilst doing a lawful act without negligence, recklessness or intent to kill or cause serious injury

- Self defence and the defence of others or property—where only such force as is reasonable has been used

Criminal homicide

Murder is the killing of a human being by a human being with malice aforethought, death occurring within a year and a day.

Manslaughter is the unlawful killing of a human being by a human being. This can be split into voluntary and involuntary manslaughter.

Voluntary manslaughter. The offender was:

- Suffering from diminished responsibility
- Provoked
- Party to a suicide pact

Involuntary manslaughter. This is where a person causes the death of another by:

- An unlawful act which carried an obvious risk of injury to another
- Doing an unlawful act recklessly
- Gross negligence to perform a duty

It is obviously a lawful act to treat a casualty and although it is hard to imagine ambulance personnel carrying out that duty recklessly it should still be understood that there is a responsibility when dealing with the life or health of another to use competent skill and sufficient attention, for if the patient dies for want of either it may be manslaughter.

In the case of the duty arising from the care or custody of a helpless person, mere negligence or inadvertence is insufficient to justify a charge of manslaughter. There must be gross negligence such as a reckless disregard of an obvious injury to health.

As in so much of the criminal and traffic law, the acid test is usually the state of mind. Ambulance personnel acting with care and with the best interest of their patient at heart cannot really go wrong.

PROPERTY

Property can be the source of many problems and an awareness of this can save ambulance personnel from a lot of trouble. There is no legal obligation on ambulance personnel to deal with property in any particular way. Accusations of misconduct and civil action can be the consequences of not dealing with property belonging to patients in a reasonable and careful manner.

There are sets of rules adopted by each service to cover the actions of their staff in relation to patients' property, and these should be observed. The following are suggestions in dealing with the subject:

- If at all possible, have nothing to do with the personal property of your patient. Where property has to be retained by anyone, let it be the police or the hospital staff.
- If it is necessary to remove items such as rings or watches in order to properly treat the patient, then let the patient keep them himself. If he is not conscious, put them in a small plastic bag and pin this conspicuously to his clothing.
- Whatever action you take with regard to property try to have a witness as to the correctness of your actions.
- When it is necessary to search a patient's property to establish identity or to locate information as to his illness, state what you are doing and why. It may reassure your patient as well as bystanders.
- Where there is other property, such as a motor vehicle, seek the assistance of the police in securing or retaining such property. If the police are not in attendance or otherwise unable to assist, then endeavour to secure the property yourself. If you can lock up a vehicle or a house and any valuables can be hidden away out of sight, you may have done as great a service to your patient as in dealing with his injury.
- If you have had to remove property from one place to another, make a note of it and seek a counter-signature from a witness.
- When you hand a patient's property to someone, obtain some form of receipt for it, even if it is only in a notebook. Make sure the receipt includes:
    1 Time and date
    2 Full name and address of the recipient
    3 Signature of the recipient
    4 Detailed list of property and its source
    5 Your own name

Time spent on safeguarding yourself in regard to other people's property is time well spent. It is better to spend 10 minutes making a detailed list rather than 10 hours explaining why you cannot account for some small item. The integrity of ambulance personnel, who have access to people's pockets and homes, must be above reproach.

DEATH

Her Majesty's Coroner and the police acting under his instruction have responsibility for all matters concerning bodies.

Where death has been certified by a doctor or has obviously occurred, the body should be left alone and responsibility handed over, preferably to a police constable. There must be continuity of evidence to show that the body at the scene is the same as that received at the mortuary. To this end, if a police constable is not available, it is preferable to have one person who can provide this evidence rather than several providing only part of it.

Dying declaration

Where a person, knowing that he is dying, makes a statement concerning the cause of his death, this may be a dying declaration. Such a statement may be used as evidence at a later date and to this end should be written down at the time or as soon as possible afterwards.

MENTAL HEALTH

The Mental Health Act (1983) allows for the compulsory admission of certain patients to hospital. An order made under the Act is enforceable by law with the help of the police if necessary.

The sections of the Act of relevance to the ambulance service are:

Section 2—admission for assessment

This allows for admission for up to 28 days and gives the right to apply to a Mental Health Review Tribunal within 14 days.

Section 3—admission for treatment

This allows for admission for up to 6 months unless the order is renewed and gives the right to apply to a Mental Health Review Tribunal within the first 6 months and once during each subsequent period.

Section 4—admission for assessment in cases of emergency

This application is made by a social worker, or the nearest relative in exceptional cases. The maximum term is 72 hours, but may be regraded (Section 2) by a second medical opinion.

Section 5—application in respect of a patient already in hospital

This allows the detention of a patient already receiving any form of inpatient treatment. It is valid for a period of up to 72 hours. Appropriately trained nurses may detain a patient for up to 6 hours whilst a doctor is found.

Section 136—emergency admissions

This allows police constables to remove to a place of safety a person whom they find in a public place who appears to be suffering from mental disorder. This can be done in the patient's own interest or for the protection of others.

FORCED ENTRY

Ambulance personnel have no right to make a forced entry into private property. Where it is necessary the assistance of the police should be sought. However, to force an entry into a house with the intention of rescuing or assisting somebody believed to be ill or injured is not burglary. Neither is it criminal damage since the Criminal Damage Act (1971) recognizes 'reasonable excuse'. Civil liability does remain.

Bibliography for Further Reading

Adams C. (1978) *Outlines of Fractures*. Edinburgh: Churchill Livingstone.

Bradley D. (1980) *Accident and Emergency Nursing*, 2nd edn. London: Baillière Tindall.

Clyne D.G.W. (1980) *A Concise Textbook for Midwives*. London: Faber and Faber.

Department of Health and Social Security (HC(78)45, December 1978).

Henry J. and Volans G. (1985) *ABC of Poisoning*. London: British Medical Association.

Jackson S. (1979) *Anatomy and Physiology for Nurses*. London: Baillière Tindall.

Mather S.J. and Edbrooke D.L. (1986) *Prehospital Emergency Care*. Bristol: Wright.

McInnes H. (1972) *International Mountain Rescue Handbook*. London: Constable.

Snook R. (1974) *Medical Aid at Accidents*. London: Update Publications.

Wilson D.H. and Hall M.H. (1979) *Casualty Officer's Handbook*. London: Butterworths.

Zorab J.S.M. and Baskett P.J.F. (1977) *Immediate Care*. Philadelphia: W.B. Saunders.

Index

Note: Page numbers in italic refer to illustrations